Case Histories in Psychiatry

Eamonn Fottrell

MD, MRCPsych, DPM
Consultant Psychiatrist, West Lambeth
Health Authority

Churchill Livingstone

EDINBURGH LONDON MELBOURNE AND NEW YORK 1983

CHURCHILL LIVINGSTONE
Medical Division of Longman Group Limited

Distributed in the United States of America by Churchill
Livingstone Inc., 1560 Broadway, New York, N.Y. 10036, and
by associated companies, branches and representatives
throughout the world.

First published 1983

ISBN 0 443 02362 X

British Library Cataloguing in Publication Data
Fottrell, Eamonn
   Case histories in psychiatry.
   1. Psychiatry — Case students
   I. Title
   616.89′09   RC465

Library of Congress Cataloging in Publication Data
   Fottrell, Eamonn.
      Case histories in psychiatry.

   Includes bibliographical references.
   1. Psychiatry — Case studies. I. Title. [DNLM:
   1. Psychiatry — Case studies. 2. Mental disorders — Case
   studies. WM 40 F761c]
   RC465.F63   1983   616.89′09   82-25512

Printed in Singapore by
Selector Printing Co Pte Ltd.

Case Histories in Psychiatry

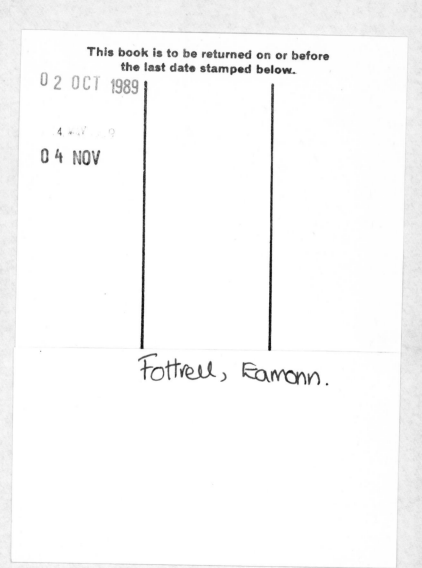

This book is to be returned on or before
the last date stamped below.

02 OCT 1989

04 NOV

Case Histories in Psychiatry

Preface

The student of psychiatry has already many textbooks to choose from. Indeed, his problem may be where to find the text with the most generally accepted view or that most likely to please the examiners. Having found his book he is tempted to espouse its view as definitive. Psychiatry is an inexact discipline in which theories abound and new knowledge is continually modifying the old. Nothing aggravates the examiner so much as the student who adopts a rigid or dogmatic view on diagnosis or management even while quoting freely from his text. In the individual patient the interaction of a psychiatric illness with his personality, which is subject to many varying influences, will in many ways be unique. Each new patient will then present a new and exciting challenge, which can only be met by a flexible response from the doctor. Many students of psychiatry are afflicted with a condition which could be described as 'The First Rank Syndrome'. This is characterised by an irrestible impulse to commit themselves to a particular diagnosis or treatment regime because a particular sign or signs were noted at some time. Psychiatric diagnoses are frequently time related and in practice one commonly finds that the diagnosis not only varies over a period, but also with the particular interviewing doctor. While diagnosis, of course, is important for orientating the psychiatrist towards the patient, emphasis in this book is on a formulation. This will include an attempt at diagnosis while summarising the interplay of relevant genetic, constitutional, social and personality factors. The case histories represent a cross section of the type of problems the doctor studying for his membership of the College of Psychiatrists must be familiar with. As psychiatric problems present with increasing frequency in general medicine, and indeed, many patients are first encountered in general medical practice, casualty, or the general practitioner's surgery, this book will be helpful to students of general medicine and doctors who do not intend to follow a career in psychiatry. The approach to management is multidisciplinary so the social worker, the psychologist, the community psychiatric nurse and the occupational therapist will also find this book valuable. Questions and discussions are centred on the patient and his problems. As this book does not claim to be definitive it is expected that many will not only disagree with the answers, but also with one another as well. Each case history is followed by a short relevant reading list with many items in the form of review articles and most are to be read in readily available journals. Reference to this reading list will place the reader in an informed position to challenge the opinions of the author and will introduce him to the ever increasing psychiatric literature of relevance to his individual patient's problems, and make him aware of the current exciting debates in the psychiatric field. This may be a remedy for textbook tediousness.

I wish to thank Dr Michael Pritchard and Dr Peter Sylvester for donating case histories and Mrs Florence Banwell for secretarial assistance.

London, 1983

E.F.

CASE 1

A 41-year-old lady is brought to hospital by the police after she was found by them undressing in the street. She is single lives alone in a flat and works as a computer programmer in a large business firm. Both parents are well, her father worked as a manager in a transport firm, she has a younger sister who is married and there is no family history of psychiatric illness. She had a happy childhood, there were no childhood neurotic traits and she left school at seventeen with two 'O' levels and one 'A' level and did a course in computer operating and programming. She has worked in this field since qualifying and has held her present post for seven years. She had the menarche at 13, her periods are regular, and she is heterosexual and has had two long relationships with men but at present has not got a boyfriend. Her interests are reading, watching television, attending the theatre, dancing and travel. Physically she is well. In the last eight years she has had four admissions to psychiatric hospitals. The first was when she was 32-years-old and she was hospitalised for four weeks and diagnosed as suffering from a 'depressive illness'. Three years later she was again hospitalised and diagnosed as suffering from a schizoaffective disorder and treated with chlorpromazine — a 100 mg O.D. and orphenadrine 50 mg t.d.s. She remained well for four years when she was readmitted and the differential diagnosis included schizophrenia or hypomania. She presented with delusions of persecution but these were in the setting of definite features of hypomania such as hyperactivity, pressure of thought, flight of ideas and elation of mood. She responded to treatment with trifluperazine 10 mg t.d.s. and was discharged on fluphenazine deconoate 25 mg I.M. every two weeks to attend a psychiatric outpatients regularly and has remained well up to the onset of her present symptoms. There is no obvious cause for the onset of her present symptoms and she was well when seen two weeks previously at outpatients. At interview she is unco-operative and incapable or unwilling to give a coherent history and claims to be mentally well, and 'on top of the world'. She denies having delusions or hallucinations or feelings of depression, and is not able to say why she went onto the street and started to strip. She exhibits flight of ideas and pressure of speech and is much more disinhibited in speech and behaviour then when she is well. She says she is going to a party and invites the doctor to accompany her. To the question, 'How do you feel?', she responds, 'All chemicals are under control, the bowels are working, are we still on biorhythms, or have we gone beyond, I could dance to a good rhythm'. She speaks in an 'upper crust' style, gesticulating frequently and gives an overall 'grandiose' impression. She has never been known to abuse drugs, she exhibits slight involuntary movements of the lips and tongue suggestive of early tardive dyskinesia.

Questions

1. What is your diagnosis?

2. What is the postulated neurophysiological basis for neuroleptic induced tardive dyskinesia?

3. What do you know in general of tardive dyskinesia?

4. What are your views on 'drug holidays' from neuroleptic medication?

5. What effects may phenothiazines have on endocrine function in premenopausal women?

6. In view of this patient's diagnostic record briefly argue in favour of the following statement 'Manic depressive psychosis and schizophrenia are not unrelated distinct clinical entities'.

7. What do you know of human leucocyte antigen (H.L.A.) research and schizophrenia?

8. How would you treat this patient?

Answers

Q1.

This patient with a history of four psychiatric admissions over a period of nine years and who has been diagnosed at different admissions as suffering from depression, from schizoaffective illness and from schizophrenia, presently exhibits florid symptomatology strongly suggestive of hypomania. She is overactive, has pressure of thought and speech, is euphoric and grandiose, exhibits, flight of ideas and is without insight into her condition. There is mild involuntary movement of her lips and tongue suggestive of early tardive dyskinesia probably induced by long term antipsychotic drug therapy. Her good response to hospitalisation and treatment in the past, suggests that at least the immediate prognosis is good, but a 'drug holiday' may be indicated in view of the presence of involuntary movements.

Q2.

A popular hypothesis is that tardive dyskinesia results from an imbalance in the postulated reciprocal relationship between dopaminergic and cholinergic neurones in the basal ganglia. Many phenothiazines are both antidopaminergic and anticholinergic. An imbalance, due to phenothiazines can result which appears to favour dopamine transmission at the expense of acetylcholine transmission, so initially a relative dopamine excess appears. This excess results from either increased dopamine turnover or from a denervation type of supersensitivity. Observations on drugs which influence dopamine action give results consistent with this hypothesis. For example phenothiazines antagonise dopamine action on synaptic receptors and often suppress the symptoms of tardive dyskinesia and drugs that directly stimulate dopamine receptors such as amphetamine and L-dopa can exacerbate the abnormal movements. Withdrawal of phenothiazines or therapy with anticholingerics for a patient with signs of tardive dyskinesia can exacerbate the abnormal movements. The early stages of tardive dyskinesia may be due to increased release of dopamine due to feedback loop stimulation in response to dopamine blockade by the phenothiazines. This form may be reversible. The later stages with denervation supersensitivity may be irreversible due to damage to the presynaptic membrane.

Q3.

Tardive dyskinesia includes orolingual dyskinesia, chorea, athetosis, dystonia, and tics but not rhythmic tremor. It may vary in intensity from isolated dyskinesias to widespread disabling dystonias which can interfere with feeding and walking. Conditions which must be considered in the differential diagnosis include stereotyped movements of schizophrenia, Huntington's chorea, Wilson's disease, rheumatic chorea and focal dystonias. The condition may be assessed with the help of the abnormal involuntary movement scale A.I.M.S. and in conjunction with a modified abbreviated dyskinesia rating scale an overall assessment of severity of symptoms can be achieved in about five minutes. An ultrasound technique for the measurement of tardive dyskinesia has also been described. Although there is a clear association between the use of anti psychotic drugs and the development of tardive dyskinesia, neither prolonged exposure nor exposure to large dosages are the determining factors in its occurrence. Older people and women appear to be at risk, and between 10 to 20 per cent of patients on antipsychotic drugs develop the condition after one year. Treatment is an exercise in balancing the risks of continuing treatment against the risks of stopping it, and has to be made on an individual basis. Withdrawal of the drugs may at least temporarily exacerbate the symptoms and treatment with amine depleting drugs such as resperine seem only temporarily effective. Treatment with acetylcholine-precursors such as choline, and lecithin remains unimpressive. Psychiatrists should try to identify patients who do not need ongoing antipsychotic medication, by observing the effects of 'drug holidays'. Some authors advocate that the prolonged use of antipsychotic drugs (over six months) is indicated only in the maintenance treatment of schizophrenia in which a continuing response can be observed, this is a controversial view.

Q4.

Although the efficacy of long term neuroleptic medication is reasonably well established, the risk of unwanted side effects is considerable. These include extrapyramidal symptoms, weight gain, the sudden death syndrome, the malignant neuroleptic syndrome of hypertonicity and hyperthermia and of course tardive dyskinesia. The object of treatment should therefore be to maintain the patient on the smallest dose of drug for the shortest possible time, which is compatible with his psychiatric well being. There is, however, little clear cut information on how long regular medication should continue for schizophrenic patients. Some authors suggest that maintenance therapy is required for at least two years. It has also been observed that patients in the community treated with long acting preparations for three to four years who defaulted had a higher relapse rate than those who continued treatment. It has not been shown with this group, however, that the defaulting group were not a poorer prognostic group than those who continued treatment and were not already beginning to relapse before they stopped treatment and some of these patients may have suffered from 'withdrawal psychosis' after prolonged neuroleptic therapy. The decision on whether a 'drug holiday' is indicated will then have to be made on an individual basis with no clear guide lines from the literature. In general schizophrenic patients with late onset psychosis and those regarded as of good prognosis may be tried. Chronic schizophrenic inpatients have the advantage of being under supervision and are at less risk than schizophrenic outpatients. Patients showing early signs of tardive dyskinesia may also merit consideration for 'drug holidays' and female patients whose illness started after the age of 40 are also reported as benefiting. There is also a latent period before relapse varying from 6–12 weeks in different reports and it would be advisable to see patients on 'drug holidays' during this period to estimate their relapse time and if they remain symptom free, the 'holiday' period could be extended by increments.

Q5.

Interest in the effects of phenothiazines on endocrine function in women was stimulated by the observation that some women develop inappropriate lactation (galactorrhoea) and/or amenorrhoea and had false positive pregnancy tests while receiving treatment with phenothiazines. These effects are thought to result mainly from the influence of phenothiazines on the endocrine regulating centre in the hypothalamus, but the precise mechanisms involved are not fully understood. On investigation plasma prolactin is found to be elevated and in amenorrhoeic patients – basal luteinising hormone values are found to be variable and cycle peaks are absent and oestrogen and progesterone levels are similar to values in the follicular stage of a normal cycle. On withdrawal of phenothiazines plasma prolactin levels fall and breast secretion diminishes. In amenorrhoeic patients withdrawal of drugs leads to resumption of a normal menstrual cycle with a normal cyclical pattern of luteinising hormone, and of oestrogens and progesterone. The raised prolactin-inhibiting values are presumably due to direct suppresion of prolactin-inhibiting factor in the hypothalamus, but there is no evidence of a general suppression of luteinising hormone releasing factor. A peripheral feed back mechanism stimulated by high levels of circulatory prolactin may be responsible for influencing luteinising hormone release.

Q6.

Probably the most cogent argument in favour of this statement is based on the lack of a universally acceptable definition of schizophrenia. The apparent frequency with which schizophrenia and manic-depressive psychosis occur together in the same patient consecutively or concurrently is far greater (up to 18 per cent) than the incidence of each illness in the general population. It is manicdepressive psychosis which causes most confusion in differentiation from 'schizophrenia'. The problem in differentiating mania from schizophrenia was evident in the findings of the U.S. — U.K. diagnostic project. Schizophrenia (even when the diagnosis is relatively clear) may be frequently accompanied by mood changes, not amounting to frank manic-depressive psychosis. It is also important to be aware that a schizophrenic-like syndrome may be a non specific clinical symptom not only in manic-depressive psychosis but in organic cerebral dysfunction, such as in temporal lobe epilepsy and drug induced states. A dimensional hypothesis for psychosis has been suggested and within this 'psychotic' dimension an individual may occasionally move on a continuum between the two psychoses. Consensus opinion in psychiatry regards the two psychoses as generally distinct while further genetic, biochemical and psychopathological evidence is awaited to confirm both their separateness and their degree of interrelatedness. Efforts to demonstrate discontinuity between schizophrenic and affective psychoses have so far ended in failure.

Q7.
There is substantial evidence from twin and family studies in favour of a genetic basis for schizophrenia, but attempts to discover genetic markers have so far been unrewarding. Studies on human leucocyte antigens (H.L.A.) carried out on schizophrenic patients and on controls represent attempts to identify such genetic markers, as studies of the H.L.A. system in disease have revealed an impressive list of associated disorders. Some researchers have found an increased incidence of certain types of H.L.A. antigens among schizophrenic patients and an increased incidence of other types of H.L.A. antigens among a sub group of patients exhibiting Schneider's first rank symptoms. Nevertheless concensus psychiatric opinion at present favours the view that such studies have so far failed to identify a genetic marker for schizophrenia and offers no firm support for either a genetic predisposition or an immunological basis to schizophrenia.

Q8.
This patient should be admitted to hospital as she is so acutely disturbed, and she may have to be detained under the provisions of the Mental Health Act. The substitution of oral antipsychotic preparations with low toxicity may be indicated, or a therapeutic trial with lithium may be justified, in view of the present symptomatology and phenothiazines could be omitted. If phenothiazines become necessary then a drug such as thioridazine which is claimed to cause fewer side effects should be prescribed in moderate to large

dosage. When the acute phase of the illness has subsided, then decisions on long term management will be made with the knowledge that the patient may be showing early signs of tardive dyskinesia. The possibility of allowing the patient a 'drug holiday' as soon as possible should be borne in mind, but the history suggests that ongoing treatment will be needed. The patient should be followed up frequently at outpatients.

Course and management

The patient responded well to thioridazine 100 mg t.d.s. and lithium 800 mg nocte after a period of three and a half weeks. She was discharged and returned to work after discharge and is followed up frequently at outpatients. Thioridazine was omitted one month after discharge.

Further reading

Asaka A, Okazaki Y, Namura I, Juji T, Miyamoto M, Ishikawa, BN 1981 Study of H.L.A. antigens among Japanese schizophrenics. Brit. J. Psychiat. 138: 498–500

Beumont P J U, Gelder M G, Friesen H G, Harris G W, MacKinnon P C B, Mandalbrote B M, Wiles D H 1974 The effects of phenothiazines on endocrine function: patients with inappropriate lactation and amenorrhoea. Brit J Psychiat 124: 413–419

British Medical Journal 1981 Leading article — Tardive dyskinesia. Brit. Med. J. 282: 1257–1258

Gibson A C 1978 'Drug holidays' for schizophrenics — are they practical for out-patients. In: Edwards G (ed) Current themes in schizophrenia, University of Southampton, Southampton, p 75–80

Kendell R E. Brockington I F 1980 The identification of disease entities and the relationship between schizophrenic and affective psychoses. Brit. J. Psychiat. 137: 324–331

Ollerenshaw D P 1973 The classification of the functional psychoses. Brit. J. Psychiat 122: 517–530

Sireling L, Paykel E S 1982 Mania. Brit. J. Hosp. Med. 27(5): 512–521

Watt D C 1982 The search for genetic linkage in schizophrenia. Brit. J. Psychiat. 140: 532–537

CASE 2

A 48-year-old man is referred to psychiatric outpatients from the cardiology department of a general hospital, because he is thought to be depressed. He is single, lives alone in a rented flat, lives on social security and has no psychiatric history. Both parents are dead, there are two other siblings both well, and there is no family history of psychiatric illness. The father was a cabinet-maker by trade. There were no childhood neurotic traits, he attended school up to the age of 16 and claims to have had a reasonably happy childhood. After leaving school he worked as a timekeeper on a building site and has had various semi-skilled clerical jobs in the building trade throughout his life. For the previous seven or eight years he has been unemployed mainly because of poor physical health. He describes himself as a friendly quiet man, with a small circle of friends, he is heterosexual and has had a few girl-friends. He is easy-going and not very ambitious. He drinks very moderately and used to be a heavy smoker up to eight or nine years previously when he ceased to smoke on medical advice. His medical history is marked, he had two myocardial infarctions, the first one nine years previously and the second three years ago. He had bypass surgery shortly after his second infarction and also had an aortic valve replacement, both procedures have been successful. However he still occasionally complains of chest pain. He also has a history of severe osteoarthritis of the hips and knees and he had one hip replacement operation and was treated with analgesics but never had steroid treatment. At interview he is a pleasant man, who walks with the help of a stick. He admits to feeling depressed over a period of two to three months and relates this to loneliness, social isolation, and worry about his health, especially about chest pain. He is kept under review by the cardiologists. There is no cognitive impairment, and no evidence of psychotic illness and he is not suicidal. His appetite is normal, there is no weight loss and in general his sleep is undisturbed but he sometimes takes nitrazepam 5 mg to get off to sleep. Most of the day he spends in his flat, but he used to attend a day centre three days weekly, but ceased to attend when he got bored with the 'basket making' type of work. His present medication is comprised of:- analgesics tabs 2 as required, anticoagulant therapy in the form of Warfarin tabs, the dose controlled by an anticoagulant clinic, glyceryl trinitrate 500 mg as required.

Questions

1. What is your formulation on this patient?

2. What do you know of personality types and cardiovascular disease?

3. Briefly what do you know of psychiatric disturbance in adults with chronic physical illness?

4. What role has the psychiatrist in the treatment of pain?

5. What do you know of steroid psychosis?

6. Do you know of any other drugs which can cause psychotic symptoms?

7. How would you treat this patient?

8. In the context of psychiatric treatment comment briefly on the statement 'Cure is mainly a function of time or the Gods, frequently the best I can do is ameliorate'.

Answers

Q1.

This patient could firstly be viewed as suffering from depression, reactive to poor physical health and loneliness. Alternatively the psychiatric aspect of his presentation may be de-emphasized and he could be regarded as exhibiting a normal mood response to considerable definite on-going stress. Both views may not be mutually exclusive as external stress is inherent in the concept of reactive depression. Also what would be regarded as a normal 'depressed' mood response to ongoing stress may take on the characteristics of depressive illness over a period of time. On the basis of the severity and duration of the stress, the absence of a psychiatric history and of a classical reactive depressive presentation, the most pragmatic conclusion would be to regard this as a normal reaction to stress. If this formulation is appropriate the alleviation of stress as far as this is possible, should improve the state of the patient.

Q2.

There is a well known view that relates personality types to cardiovascular disease especially coronary artery disease. According to this view individuals can be divided into two broad personality types — types A and B. Type A personalities are described as 'driven by the urgency of time pressure', are extremely competitive and if frustrated may become extremely hostile. Overall they present the picture of the ambitious hard driving executive. Easy-going individuals who are just the opposite to type A are labelled type B. Coronary artery disease was found to have twice the incidence in type A as in type B. More recently this view has been modified — there is some evidence that 'frustrated clerks and brow beaten middle management', may be at greater risk of stress induced coronary heart disease. It is thought that type A traits have been over emphasised as coronary risk factors. Individuals who over-react to stress, 'silent hyperreactors' not necessarily with type A traits, may be most vulnerable to coronary artery disease.

Q3.

The successful management of acute illness has produced a growing population with chronic illness, for whom there is not a complete cure. There is little doubt that chronic physical illness is a major cause of psychiatric disorder and related psychological disturbance of some degree is probably the rule. This may in turn result in further physical disability and dependence. For example, as many post-coronary patients fail to return to work because of social and psychological factors as for reasons of cardiac damage. Depression and anxiety states are common in these patients. The psychological disturbance will be influenced by the severity of the physical illness, the personality of the individual and the degree of medical, social, financial and familial support. One must also distinguish between the direct cerebral consequences of disease as observed in organic cerebral conditions and the indirect effect of the appreciation by the individual of deterioration in appearance and abilities. Both aspects of chronic illness may be psychiatrically deleterious and operative for example in Huntington's chorea or multiple sclerosis. Illnesses affecting sensory input may alter psychological functioning considerably as may rapidly progressive 'chronic' illness when the time for mental adaptation is not sufficient. The personality of the individual may be the determining factor in his response to illness. Illness may provide gratification of his dependency needs for the passive dependent individual and the illness may satisfy the need for punishment in the guilt ridden masochistic personality.

The familial response to the 'sick role' will also have a psychological impact on the patient. Overprotectiveness by the family and emphasis on the loss of a familial role and responsibility by the patient may have a deleterious effect. Interpersonal relationships may be threatened by the illness particularly sexuality. Sexual dysfunction may arise from psychological reaction to the illness, for example from loss of self-esteem in amputees or hemiplegics. Sexual function may be directly disturbed in endocrinological and neurological conditions and this may be very traumatic psychologically, although frequently doctors fail to inquire into this. Loss of earnings by the 'bread winner' will obviously be a cause of considerable stress and anguish, especially where health care is financially orientated. Physicians are unsure how they should respond to a patient who fails to make progress or is dying and the patients's sense of hopelessness may be reflected and reinforced by the doctor's tendency to withdraw from personal contact. Nurses may tend to respond with overprotectiveness and this may re-inforce a patient's feeling of helplessness. There is obviously a need not only to diagnose the patient but to be aware of his psychological, financial, social and personal vulnerabilities.

Q4.

Pain is an experience whose degree is determined by both the physical and emotional state of the patient. The psychiatrist will be involved in the treatment of pain not only among psychiatric patients but also among general medical and surgical patients where the emotional control of, or reaction to, pain is marked. Among psychiatric inpatients the incidence of pain in the symptomatology may be as high as 20 per cent, and 50 per cent of other psychiatric patients may have pain as one of their complaints. Chronic pain due to neurotic illness or personality disorder is very common. In general hospitals psychiatrists will see patients in whom chronic pain from an organic condition is making them feel wretched and in whom emotional factors magnify the pain. These patients will most likely be encountered in specialised pain clinics or departments of neurology, rheumatology, or in centres specialising in treating cancer. Chronic organic pain may result in personality change, behaviour disorder, anxiety, depression, irritability and resentment in the sufferer. The psychiatrist may not only get involved in the direct treatment of pain, but also in the treatment of its psychological effects. Treatment is essentially that of the underlying disorder. Adequate but not excessive investigation of possible physical causes is required. Success may be obtained by all techniques when appropriate — these include psychotherapy, antidepressants, behaviour therapy, placebos, marital therapy, attention distraction relaxation therapy, phenothiazines, biofeedback techniques and of course discreet use of analgesics.

Q5.

Although steroids were regarded as among the 'wonder drugs' of the late 1940's and are very useful in a variety of conditions, they have significant adverse effects and among these is psychosis. This is now accepted as a definite risk of therapy. This adverse effect is not surprising when one considers the depressed mood frequently found in both Addison's disease and Cushing's syndrome. The exact mechanism of induction of the psychosis is unknown but it is thought that exogenous steroids and A.C.T.H. disrupt the hypothalamic pituitary adrenal axis. Warning symptoms of steroid psychosis include frontal paraesthesias of the head, insomnia and restlessness. Most patients with steroid psychosis present in a manic fashion with flight of ideas, pressure of speech, grandiose ideation, lack of inhibition and judgement which may result in buying sprees, foolish business management, and reckless driving. When thwarted the patient becomes angry and aggressive. There may be associated delusions and auditory hallucinations. Depression with suicidal ideation may sometimes be the presenting feature. The incidence varies with the preparation and the dosage, for example with prednisone the incidence varies from 1 per cent at low dosage to 18 per cent with high dosage. Onset of psychosis is usually delayed to about the third or the fourth week of therapy. The absence of a psychiatric history does not guarantee immunity, and a history of psychiatric illness does not necessarily contraindicate therapy, although an underlying affective disorder may be unmasked during treatment. Treatment consists primarily of omitting or reducing the steroid and of the introduction of antipsychotic medication in appropriate dosage. Hospitalisation may be indicated for the very disturbed patient, for his own protection.

Q6.

Among drugs which can cause psychotic symptoms are included — alcohol, barbiturates, sympathomimetic amines, disulfiram, isoniazid, bromides, L-dopa, anticholinergics, benzodiazepines, hallucinogens and L.S.D. A drug history obtained from the patient or others may be very important in assessing altered mental functioning.

Q7.

Arrangements should be made for this patient to attend a psychiatric day hospital, where further observation and assessment could continue. This would also ensure that he has a social outlet at least on a few occasions weekly. It may be appropriate as he improves to refer him on to an assessment cum rehabilitation centre with a view to eventually finding sheltered employment or at least attending an industrial therapy centre where there would be a variety of work available. Should the patient not improve mentally then it would be necessary to consider antidepressant therapy and its effects should be closely monitored due to his medical history. With social rehabilitation the psychiatric prognosis may be reasonably bright.

Q8.

In the psychiatric context this statement could be interpreted as emphasing the limitations of psychiatric treatment. Schizophrenic and manic depressive patients are frequently maintained or helped rather than cured by therapy. Antidepressant therapy may commonly be unsuccessful or patients may readily relapse. Neurotic patients may require many years of therapy before improvement appears as may many patients described as personality disordered or psychopathic. For those who abuse or are dependent on alcohol or drugs, a successful outcome is more often dependent on the insight and motivation of the patient than on the exertions of the psychiatrist. There is at present no method of halting or slowing up the brain failure processes so common in the elderly. However, many illnesses both psychiatric as well as medical result either from poor genetic endowment or predisposition, are the end product of unhealthy life styles or adverse social circumstances or are indicative of degenerative processes, or combinations of these factors. Few illnesses are 'cured' solely by the doctor and always require an endogenous healing response even in the case of a minor surgical procedure, to compliment the exogenous effort of the doctor. To the degree that this endogenous response is lacking, most frequently will the efforts of the doctor be unsuccessful. Although the treatment of the psychiatrist may be infrequently curative, there is little doubt that psychiatric intervention can ameliorate and shorten the duration of acute symptoms of many illnesses, such as depression and schizophrenia. By the use of a multidisciplinary team, the psychiatrist not only recognises his limitations in dealing with all aspects of psychiatric illness but in those conditions in which time is the main healer such as personality disorders and neurotic states, tries to ensure that the illness will not be over traumatic for the patient or his family. The degree of support available from a psychiatric service to a motivated drug or alcohol dependent patient can determine final success or failure, and a well organised psychogeriatric service can at least provide care for a 'brain failure' patient and alleviate considerably the burden on relatives.

Course and management

The patient attended a day hospital daily for three weeks and was then referred to a rehabilitation assessment unit. He improved considerably over a period of five weeks and psychotropic medication was not needed and arrangements were made for him to do sheltered work in an industrial therapy setting.

Further reading

Davies M H 1981 Stress personality and coronary artery disease. Brit J Hosp Med. 26(4): 350–360

Falk E 1981 Steroid psychosis, diagnosis and treatment. In: Manchrenk T C (ed) Psychiatric Medicine update, 1981 edn, Churchill Livingstone, Edinburgh, London, Melbourne, p 147–153

Kornfeld J 1981 Hypereactors not Type A's — highest cardiovascular risk. Medical News (11 June): 14–15

Merskey H 1980 Psychiatry and the treatment of pain. Brit J Psychiat 136: 600–602

Taylor P 1978 psychological disturbance in adults with chronic physical illness. In: Gaind R N, Hudson B L (eds) Current themes in psychiatry, Macmillan Press Ltd, London and Basingstoke

CASE 3

A consultant psychiatrist is asked to do a domiciliary consultation by a general practitioner, on a 73-year-old man. He is living alone and is reported to be confused, and verbally aggressive, to be uncooperative with community support facilities, and at risk living in the community. The history is obtained mainly from the general practitioner and the local social services personnel who know him well. There is no psychiatric history. He refuses to volunteer any information about his parents, his childhood or early teenage years. All his life he has worked as a plasterer and he got married in 1930 shortly before the birth of their only child, a son. The marital relationship quickly deteriorated and he was eventually separated and divorced and the son was reared by his wife and he has had no contact with the son or wife since. He is described as a decisive man, eccentric, occasionally dressing flamboyantly, inclined to readily write complaining letters to the local papers, and to 'pester' his general practitioner. There are few if any close friends and his main social outlet is when he attends church and a local church organisation. Because of arthritis of the hips and knees he hasn't worked for the last 12 years and has been wheel-chair bound for the last year and a half. His accommodation is comprised of the ground floor flat of a late Victorian semi-detached two-story house, the upper flat is unoccupied. He has a kitchen, bathroom with toilet, two bedrooms and a reception room and he is the proprietor. Up to recently he had a home help who did cleaning, shopping and cooking, and a volunteer from the church visiting five times weekly, but in the last week he threw an ashtray at the home help and was abusive and exposed his genitalia to the volunteer and they have ceased visiting. A meals on wheels service is provided seven days weekly, and he is at risk when he turns on the gas and forgets to light it. He leaves his front door open and youths have stolen some of his property, vandalised some more and written slogans on the wall in the hall. The home is untidy and his food is comprised mainly of bread and tea and a considerable quantity of unwashed crockery is evident. On examination the patient is in a wheelchair which he can manipulate with ease, and he appears to be in good nutritional state. He is abrupt in his replies, resents the visit, and reluctantly answers questions. He denies feeling depressed, exhibits a mood of anger rather than depression. It is evident that he has some cognitive impairment. His sleeping pattern appears to be undisturbed. His recall of information is slow, but he can give his address, knows his general practitioner's name and the road he lives on, but

knows little of current affairs and has difficulty in naming the present monarch and the prime minister. He has great difficulty in
retaining new information. He indicts community support facilities
by saying, 'they only come to see what they can get out of me,
they don't care about me'; otherwise there are no psychiatric features evident. He is not suicidal. His present medication is comprised of thioridazine 25 mg t.d.s., nitrazepam one tab nocte,
indomethacin one capsule t.d.s. He has a long history of arthritis
for which treatment has consisted mainly of analgesics. Otherwise
he is physically well.

Questions

1. What is your formulation on this patient?

2. How would you obtain a psychiatric history on a reluctant historian like this patient?

3. How do differing psychiatric interviewing techniques compare?

4. What problems do the elderly mentally infirm present to health
   and social services?

5. What do you know of sexual deviation in the elderly?

6. Is there a relationship between social class and admission rates
   to psychiatric hospitals?

7. What are the indications for hospitalisation of the elderly mentally ill?

8. What advice would you give to a nurse who complains about
   an elderly demented patient, 'Everytime I go near he grabs me
   by the breast'?

Answers

Q1.
Within the limits of information available on this patient, he probably is suffering with incipient dementia characterised by cognitive
impairment which is difficult to classify. In conjunction with this

he appears to have a paranoid aggressive behaviour disorder characterised by abusive and threatening language. His physical incapacity and his behaviour have resulted in social isolation which in turn tends to exacerbate his behaviour disorder. His previous personality pattern is unknown but there is a suggestion that he may have been a hypersensitive, easily offended, if not frankly paranoid type of person. At present he is at risk from self-neglect, from fire or explosions, and from intruders. Hospitalisation for further assessment and to initiate long term planning is indicated.

Q2.

A very informative history may be elicited from a reluctant historian, by establishing rapport with him and gaining his confidence, by a series of discussions and interviews over a period of time. It will become clear to the patient that the object of the questioning is to ascertain his particular needs, and his vulnerabilities so that he can be helped. Collateral histories from general practitioners, social workers and relatives will not only help to complete the history, but may disclose particular aspects which the patient considers unimportant, and which may be crucial to diagnosis and management.

Q3.

There are differing views among clinicians on the most effective means of obtaining valid factual information for diagnostic purposes. Some advocate a comprehensive series of standard questions to ensure that all relevant information is obtained. Some state that this is not sufficient as replies in first interviews may be ambiguous or contradictory. It has been suggested by others that probing and cross questioning is needed to get a precise picture of events and behaviour. Structured clinical type interviews, however, have been criticised on the basis that they generate resistance in the patient and in collateral interviewees. It is also suggested that the patient is in the most advantageous position to appreciate the most meaningful topics for him, and he will direct attention to them in a less structured interview. The mere collection of factual data may take precedence in a formal structured interview over the establishment of a personal therapeutic relationship between the doctor and the patient. There is general agreement that an accurate diagnostic formulation requires a great deal of factual information of a clinical, social and familial kind. The experienced interviewer should not have undue difficulty in reconciling the need for factual information with the therapeutic doctor patient relationship so necessary in successful psychiatric treatment, especially if the doctor patient contact is ongoing over a period.

Q4.

Elderly mentally infirm patients, not only because of their multiple infirmities but particularly because of brain failure, present perhaps the biggest challenge to health and social services for the foreseeable future. It is estimated that 1 in 10 old people over the age of 65 in the United Kingdom is suffering from some degree of dementia and approximately 14 per cent of the population is now in this age category. Thus with these figures in a catchment area district of 200 000 there would be 28 000 over the age of 65 and 2 800 of these would have some degree of dementia. The size of this 65 + population is expected to increase to 16 per cent in the 1990s and then level off. The population of 'old old' that is those aged 75 and upwards is expected to go on increasing even when the overall number of 65-year-olds levels off. They are expected to increase by 35 per cent in the next 20 years. This population will make exceedingly great demands on health and social services. Two thirds of them will be women, mainly single or widowed and of course it is in this group that the dementing illnesses and problems of emotional and physical dependency have their highest incidence. Handicapping memory defects have been found in 50 per cent of people over 85 and 20 per cent of people over 80 suffer from incapacitating mental deterioration. Mental changes severely jeopardise self care in a third of subjects aged 90 or more. Approximately 50 per cent of the population of mental hospitals is over 65 years and at least 50 to 60 per cent of these will suffer with dementia. Also patients who have grown old in hospital, 'graduates', have serious difficulties in self care such as incontinence, dressing, dyspraxia, mobility and feeding difficulties. These patients require a high nursing ratio, and most psychiatric hospitals are chronically short of nurses. Hospital managers have tried to cope by re-allocating resources within psychiatric hospitals but satisfactory solutions are rarely found, due primarily to serious under financing. The present level of residential and sheltered accommodation in the community is quite inadequate to cope with the population of patients not needing hospitalisation. Local authorities are unable to finance an adequate home help, social worker and meals on wheels service to facilitate community service.

Q5.

Sexual deviation is not uncommon in the elderly, especially the elderly male. With ageing there may be a reduction in the cortical controlling influences and inhibition. Covert sexual behaviour may become overt. The most common deviations encountered are exhibitionism and paedophilia and these are very rarely accompanied by violence. Dementia is the commonest psychiatric condition associated with sexual deviation in the elderly, more rarely affective disturbance may be an associated factor. Many elderly deviants are of course just young deviants grown old and there may be a history of personality disorder or of involvement with the law.

Q6.

There is a relationship between social class and admission rates to psychiatric hospitals for the elderly. Studies in the United States have shown that 4/5 of admissions of patients aged 65 and upwards to psychiatric hospitals occurred in the lower income group. Many of these patients are found to be living alone, or with unrelated persons, or in run-down areas where there is an increased risk of physical assault. Lack of financial and family support and limited access to services and friends exacerbate existing psychiatric states. Elderly blacks have a disproportionate amount of major psychiatric illnesses and are over represented in the lower social groups and among the underprivileged. The high social groups are, of course, more financially secure, have more familial support, live in pleasant surroundings and when psychiatrically ill may be maintained privately at home or in nursing homes.

Q7.

An elderly psychiatrically ill person should be admitted to hospital, when adequate treatment in the community is impossible because of non-compliance or unsuitable setting and/or when he represents a danger to himself or others and it is likely that improvement cannot be expected while he remains in the community. As far as possible hospitalisation should be avoided as it may result in increased agitation, depression and confusion. There is also the danger that a medically ill patient who has prominent psychiatric symptomatology may be misplaced in a psychiatric ward and receive less than optimum medical care. In practice patients with depression and suicidal ideas, those with severe organic brain disease who cannot be maintained at home, alcohol and drug abusers who need detoxification, and those with chronic severe psychoses whose medication needs adjustment and regulation, are most frequently in need of hospitalisation. Hospitalisation may also be necessary for patients for whom community support facilities of various kinds have been unsuccessful such as some with brain failure and whose existence in the community is characterised by an on-going series of psychiatric and social crises. Hospitalisation may also be necessary to render 'holiday relief' to caring relatives and to assess appropriateness for various forms of long term care.

Q8.

An elderly demented person may behave like this when behavioural inhibiting influences are reduced. It could also be indicative of a need for warmth and personal contact which is a perfectly normal need. This need may not be readily satisfied in the setting of a psychiatric ward. Avoiding or reprimanding the person for his inappropriate behaviour is unlikely to be successful as it does not satisfy his need. The most appropriate response may be to take the patient's hand and stroke it or put an arm around his shoulder while talking to him, this will fulfil to some degree his need for human contact.

Course and management

The patient was admitted to hospital informally where he was found to be suffering from early dementia, thought to be predominately multi-infarct in type, in the setting of a sensitive somewhat paranoid personality. He behaved well in hospital, psychotropic medication was not needed. He was discharged after six weeks to a residential home for the elderly on the condition that should he misbehave and become a problem for the home then re-admission to hospital would be considered.

Further reading

Arie T, Isaacs A D 1978 The development of psychiatric services for the elderly in Britain. In: Isaacs, Post (ed) Studies in geriatric psychiatry, John Wiley and Sons, Chichester, New York, Brisbane, Toronto, p 241–261

Cox A, Rutter M, Holbroak D 1981 Psychiatric interviewing techniques V. Experimental study: eliciting factual information. Brit J Psychiat 139: 29–37

Tennent T G 1981 Antisocial sexual deviations. Smith, Kline and French Publications Ltd Booklet, ESD Printing and Binding Ltd, London

CASE 4

A 30-year-old woman is brought to outpatients of a psychiatric hospital by the police. They were called to see her because she had to be restrained from getting onto the rails in a tube station. She states that she wishes to kill herself. She was born and reared in Britain and describes her parents as 'working class' and attended school up to the age of 16. She was near the top of her class and claims to have had a happy childhood and she has two younger siblings. There were no childhood neurotic traits. The parents and the siblings are well and there is no psychiatric history among her relatives. After leaving school she worked as a shop assistant and subsequently as a factory worker for six years and then got married to a factory porter. The marriage was described as 'stormy' and the husband accused her of having 'affairs' which she denies and they were divorced after four years. There is one daughter aged seven who is cared for by the patient's mother. For the preceding three years she had worked mainly at domestic work but at present is unemployed. She is sharing a 'bed-sit' with a girl friend, she is heterosexual, smokes 30 cigarettes daily, drinks moderately and likes to 'visit the pub with my friend when we can afford it'. Her interests are in 'modern music, television, and clothes'. She has no boy friend at present. She keeps in contact with her daughter by visiting her a couple of times a year, but she describes her relationship with her parents as 'cool', meaning by this that they are critical of her and somewhat rejecting. There is a history of one psychiatric admission for the treatment of depression and a mild overdose of tricyclic antidepressants shortly after she was divorced. She claims to have been reasonably well since. For the preceding two to three weeks she has felt depressed and lonely especially when her friend goes out to work. There is, however, no disturbance in sleep or appetite and she feels well when in the company of others or when in a 'pub'. She also complains of having 'fits' in the last couple of weeks. Overall she has had three 'fits', she claims to lose consciousness, but does not bite or wet herself. Her previous medical history is negative. At interview she appears to suffer more from social isolation and loneliness than from depression. She still admits to feeling suicidal and relates this to the loss of the company of her ex-husband and relative separation from her daughter and her inability to get a suitable job. She worries about the effect that separation from her natural parents will have on her daughter and whether it will affect her psychologically. There are no psychotic features evident and she appears to be of good average intelligence and there is no history of involvement with the police or of a psychopathic behaviour disorder. Because of suicidal risk and to clarify the nature of the 'fits' the patient was admitted to hospital. Physical examination was negative, as were E.E.G. and brain scan and nursing observation of a 'fit' described an atypical clonic seizure.

Questions

1. What is your formulation on this patient?

2. What contribution does the E.E.G. make to psychiatric diagnosis?

3. What do you know of cerebral laterality and psychopathology?

4. Comment briefly on the statement 'hysteria is not only a delusion but also a snare'.

5. What determines the choice of symptoms in hysteria?

6. How would you treat this patient?

7. Briefly what effect has psychiatric illness in a parent on the children of the family?

8. What is not essential to psychotherapy?

Answers

Q1.

This patient's problem would appear mainly to be one of social isolation and loneliness. Negative aspects of her personality structure are exacerbated and accentuated by this isolation. In view of the knowledge that there does not appear to be an organic basis to her 'fits' and their atypical form it is likely that they are hysterical in nature and may represent a cry for attention and help. Her 'suicidal' attempt carried out in a public setting may be similarly motivated. Unemployment would be a further stress, not only of a financial kind but would deprive her of the companionship of colleagues and instil a sense of rejection.

Q2.

At present psychiatric diagnoses are made primarily by history taking, by mental assessment, by observation both at the time of examination and over a period of time and by the help of collateral information from family, relatives and para medical personnel. The E.E.G. may be helpful in confirming clinical impressions or shedding light on aspects of a patient's presentation, such as in this case, those presenting with 'fits', those in delirious or confused states, and those with symptoms suggesting neurological pathology. In confused states the E.E.G. is slowed and shows theta activity. In coma the slow activity progresses to a dominant delta rhythm. In senile dementia there is slowing of the alpha rhythm. In general, the E.E.G.'s are normal in neuroses and personality disorders, however, psychopathic and criminal personalities may have immature E.E.G. readings. Up to 50 per cent of schizophrenic patients may have abnormal E.E.G.'s but these are non-specific and may include low voltage fast records, or immature records with bilateral temporal theta activity. Psychotropic drugs such as major and minor tranquillisers and antidepressants may influence the E.E.G. Chlorpromazine has epileptogenic properties and in susceptible individuals and in epileptics will precipitate epileptic discharges. Amitriptyline may have similar effects and both it and chlorpromazine have been used to activate E.E.G.'s in the investigation of epilepsy. Benzodiazepines, however, may mask epileptic discharges and produce a normal record in an epileptic patient and cause confusion in investigations on the nature of 'fits' in psychiatric patients.

Q3.

By psychiatric cerebral laterality is meant a disorder, absolute or relative in function between the cerebral hemispheres which results in psychiatric illness. Interest in cerebral laterality and psychiatric illness is a relatively new and exciting line of inquiry. It has been observed using computer tomography that normally occurring lateral asymmetries in the frontal and occipital lobes were reversed more often in schizophrenics than in controls. An association between abnormal lateralization and schizophrenia has been observed in the handedness of twins. When both twins were dextral, concordance for schizophrenia was 93 per cent, but if one twin was sinistral the concordance dropped to 23 per cent, and left handed schizophrenics had a milder form of illness. Deficiencies in the integration and processing of visual, auditory and tactile stimuli between the cerebral hemispheres have also been reported in schizophrenia and it is also suggested that there is a disorder of interhemispheric communication. Regarding affective disorders there are two rival views. One suggests that mania and depression are a result of right hemisphere dysfunction, and the other suggests emotional polarity between the hemispheres with negative emotions and depressions predominating on the right side and elation and mania predominating on the left side, when there is interhemispheric imbalance. Psychopathic and neurotic disorders have also been associated with a disturbance of lateralisation. Many commentators regard some of the conclusions on psychiatric illness and laterality as simplistic and suggest that more complex models are now needed. The field of study is still in its infancy and it is unlikely that diagnostic or therapeutic break throughs will result in the immediate future, nevertheless it is leading to insights into the workings of the normal brain.

Q4.

The implications of this statement are that hysteria is a misleading diagnosis, easily arrived at, and that it is dangerous in the sense that it may lead to disastrous under investigation of a patient with organic pathology. A similar statement on hysteria is that the hysteric is the patient who has not been fully investigated. Hysteria has always eluded concise clear definition, yet it has always been with us and waxes and wanes in popularity with the medical profession. It is a time related diagnosis in that its form and presentation varies over the years. The swooning behaviour of young Victorian ladies, has long been replaced by the monoplegic, amnesic or overbreathing presentations of today. Research in the mid 1960's which demonstrated underlying physical pathology in a large percentage of patients diagnosed as hysterics, challenged the validity of the diagnosis and devalued the concept. This research however was carried out on a highly unusual series of patients with obscure neurological conditions and the conclusions arrived at were not fully justified. Since then although hysteria as a diagnosis has regained considerable respect, the present tendency is to view it as part of a symptom complex. It is an attempt, never fully conscious and frequently unconscious by the patient, to obtain relief from unmanageable stress. The patient's previous personality, his history of coping with stress, his social background, his intellectual level, the degree of stress, are all studied in an effort to make the patient's presentation more meaningful to the psychiatrist. This stress may take many forms and may include worry and anxiety over underlying physical illness or severe pain emanating from such illness. Underlying physical illness as a stressful factor resulting in a hysterical response, is intelligible and physical illness and hysteria are not mutually exclusive.

Q5.
The choice of symptoms will depend largely on the patient's knowledge and concept of common current illnesses regarded as 'respectable' by the medical profession. These will be symptoms of illnesses he has either had himself, or seen in relatives or friends or has read about. Today's popular hysterical symptoms include headaches, stomachaches and backaches. Symbolism and gain will also be determining factors. The meaning of symbolism of symptoms in hysteria is two fold. The more superficial meaning is that it is a form of 'body language', for example the hysterical paraplegic may be bringing attention to his plight by saying 'I haven't got a leg to stand on'. The deeper meaning of symbolism of symptoms may be difficult to find and may be related to unconscious problems associated with infantile sexuality. Examples of this type of symbolism are found in the writings of Freud. The role of the gain or reward factor in determining symptoms may sometimes be obvious. For example the reluctant school boy may best avoid school by symptoms relating to his feet or legs, and the recalcitrant soldier may complain of paralysis of the trigger finger. The ultimate choice of symptoms will represent the final common pathway of interaction and compromise at various levels of consciousness between all the above factors. Determining which are the more important factors in the individual case may be difficult, but intriguing.

Q6.
Treatment should be guided by the observation that the patient's suicidal behaviour and her 'fits' are probably cries for help from a person under considerable stress. The stresses influencing her appear to be comprised of loneliness and social isolation, a feeling of rejection and failure due to unemployment, and worry about the future of her daughter. Rejection and criticism by her parents may also be an adverse psychological influencing factor. Psychotropic drugs are probably not indicated, at least recourse should not be had to them initially. If the suicidal danger subsides then the patient should be discharged from hospital as soon as possible. Various treatment programmes alone or in combination may be appropriate, and only observation over a period of time will indicate which is most effective. Attendance at an industrial therapy unit with guidance and help to gain employment may be indicated. Ongoing individual supportive or group psychotherapy may be helpful to

enable the patient to clearly identify her problems and respond in a positive adaptive way to them. It may be advisable if the patient is agreeable to involve the parents even at a distance in a treatment programme to encourage mutual understanding and tolerance, and more frequent contact with her daughter should be encouraged. The prognosis will depend largely on the patient's motivation and insight and on the reserves of positive personality features.

Q7.

There is considerable evidence that psychological illness in a parent is associated with psychological disturbance in the children of the family. The severity of the parent's illness, however, is not related to the likelihood of psychological problems in the children. Children of psychotic parents are less likely to show psychological disturbance than children of parents with personality disturbance. The explanation for this may be that the psychotic parent's illness is likely to be episodic whereas the personality disordered parent may have an on-going disorder, especially during the early formative years of the children. It is the extent to which the parent and the children and the parents themselves get on badly together rather than the presence of psychiatric illness that determines the degree of disturbance in the children. The presence of a well parent will be of considerable help in counterbalancing the effects on the children of a psychologically ill parent, as may proximate and ready access to caring grandparents.

Q8.

Many misunderstandings on psychotherapy have arisen because of an artificial superstructure built around it. Psychotherapy is not comprised of a rigid set of rules which must be strictly adhered to by therapist and patient. Psychotherapy is not silence, or sitting inactively for long periods waiting for a patient to take responsibility for himself, to put no challenge or pressure on a patient is not a basic requirement of psychotherapy, nor can it rest on any limited theoretical base. Psychotherapy should not maintain that any single theory, such as trauma during birth, sexual inhibition or incestous conflict is accountable for the numerous troubles the patient may present with. Psychotherapists may be more gainfully employed in seeking for a myriad of causes rather than for one. Its practice must not be exclusive to any one group or to adherents of a particular school of thought.

Course and management

The patient was discharged from hospital after two weeks and attended an industrial therapy unit. She got a job doing domestic work shortly afterwards, attends psychiatric outpatients regularly and is not receiving psychotropic drugs. There have been no 'fits' over a four month period and the patient did not wish the parents to know of her hospitalisation or be included in a treatment programme.

Further reading

Greben S E 1981 The essence of psychotherapy. Brit J Psychiat 138: 449–455

Gruzelier J H 1981 Cerebral laterality and psychopathology. Editorial. Psychological medicine II: 219–227

Rutter M L 1966 Children of sick parents : an environmental and psychiatric study. Maudesley Monograph 16, Oxford University Press, Oxford

Sim M, Gordon E B 1976 The E E G in psychiatry. In: Basic psychiatry, 3rd edn, Churchill Livingstone, Edinburgh, London. New York p 70–76

Slater E 1965 Diagnosis of hysteria. Brit Med J 1: 1395–1399

Smith A C 1978 Hysteria. In: Gaind R N, Hudson B L (eds) Current themes in psychiatry, MacMillan Press Ltd, London and Basingstoke, p 125

CASE 5

A young man, physically robust, is brought to hospital by the police, having been found by them semi-clothed, shouting and behaving in a bizarre way on a street. On arrival in hospital he appears to be quite psychotic, is inaccessible to questioning, is very noisy and threatening and has to be physically restrained. He is tranquillised with 150 mg of chlorpromazine intra-muscularly. There are no accompanying relatives and the police have no further information on him. Physical examination is negative and the patient is detained in hospital under the provisions of the mental health act. He is treated with chlorpromazine 200 mg six hourly for the succeeding three days during which time he becomes more tranquil and accessible to questioning and volunteers personal details. He is 27-years old, a student of economics in his final year of study, is unmarried and lives with his parents. There are two older brothers in the family and there is no family history of psychiatric illness. His early childhood years and his time in primary school are unremarkable and he claims to have always been 'in the upper half of the class in exams'. After achieving one 'A' level and three 'O' levels he worked for 18 months as a representative for a drug firm, before entering college to study economics. His study has been interrupted on three previous occasions by his psychiatric illness and on each occasion he needed to be hospitalised. His social outlets are comprised mainly of reading, watching documentaries on television, playing tennis and hockey, he drinks moderately and does not smoke. He is heterosexual and has a girlfriend with whom he has associated for over two years. There is no relevant medical history and he had his first admission to a psychiatric hospital at the age of 21 'for treatment of hypomania' which responded to treatment and he was well for about 15 months when he relapsed. This again responded to hospitalisation and treatment and he remained well for about two and a half years. His last relapse was about nine months previously and he was discharged from hospital after four weeks and took lithium 1000 mg nocte and chlorpromazine 50 mg t.d.s. and attended outpatients. There is no history of depression or of the patient abusing drugs and he describes himself in a grandiose fashion as very friendly with lots of friends and says he is 'very busy developing economic theories to solve this country's ills'. The parents say that he is unreliable with taking his medication, and that he was fairly well up to 10 days previously when he refused to take any more medication claiming that it was making him drowsy and he did not need it. Subsequently he became more active physically, more talkative and argumentative, spent most of the day out of the house and began to sleep poorly. He smashed the parents' telephone after the operator refused to comply with his request to reverse charges on a call he wished to make to his girlfriend who was abroad. After this incident the parents did not see him until they were informed two days later that he had been admitted to hospital. On mental assessment three days after admission the patient is much more tranquil and accessible. However, he is still very loquacious and argumentative and gesticulates to emphasise particular points, and there is marked flight of ideas evident. The speech context is of a grandiose kind and revolves around the contribution he intends making to solve the economic ills of the world. His mood is elated. He remains insightless, feels there is no need to be in hospital and says he takes his medication 'just to keep the parents happy'. There is no clouding of consciousness, perceptual or cognitive disturbance evident and he appears to be well within the average intellectual range.

Questions

1. What is your formulation on this patient?

2. Do you know of the development of any biological tests which may help both to differentiate between the affective disorders and may indicate the appropriate treatment?

3. Write a brief comment on the statement 'Unipolar manic depressive illness is inherited differently to bipolar illness!.

4. What do you understand by the term 'mixed affective states'?

5. Do you know of any rating scale suitable for assessing this patient's hypomania?

6. How would you treat this patient?

7. Has parenteral medication an advantage over oral medication in bringing acute florid psychiatric states under control?

Answers

1.
This patient with a history of hypomania is most likely suffering from a relapse into hypomania, characterised by elation of mood,

flight of ideas, increased psychomotor activity, loss of insight and inhibition resulting in socially disruptive behaviour. There is no evidence of drug abuse. The onset of his symptoms is possibly associated with his refusal to continue his medication, but it is difficult to exclude the possibility that non-compliance with treatment might itself be symptomatic of his impending relapse. It is most likely that he will again respond to hospitalisation and treatment but a further relapse is probable.

2.

There has been a long theoretical association of affective disturbance with abnormality of the hypothalamic pituitary adrenal axis. Investigations of this association appear to be leading to the development of biological tests useful for the classification of affective disorders and for indicating appropriate treatment. For example it has been found that major endogenous depressive disorders, as distinct from reactive depressions are associated with hypersecretion of cortisol which cannot be suppressed by administration of dexamethasone in 50 per cent of cases. It is not clear why suppression occurs in half or whether the suppressed or unsuppressed half represent a particular sub type of depression responsive to a particular treatment regime. It has also been observed that patients with unipolar endogenous depression show a decreased or absent response while those with bipolar (manic-depressive) depression show an augmented response to thyrotrophin-releasing hormone. In the manic phase of bipolar illness the response to thyrotrophin-releasing hormone changes from augmented to blunted. It has been observed further that low pre-treatment serum concentrations of 3 methoxy–4-hydroxyphenylglycol among depressives is associated with a favourable response to imipramine and a failure to respond to amitriptyline and conversely for high pre-treatment levels. A scheme, although still in its very early stages, would appear to be available for the laboratory investigation of patients with affective disturbance. It may now be practical with laboratory help to separate in many cases reactive from endogenous depressions and divide those with endogenous depression into unipolar and bipolar groups. Guidance from the laboratory on the appropriate type of medication may also be forthcoming. It must be kept in mind that these tests are being developed from recent experimental findings and are not sufficiently established to justify routine use and they are intrusive and expensive. The debate on the vexed question of the continuum or the bimodal model for depressive illness continues and the problems of measurement standardisation and replication of research findings in depressive illness is the background against which these tests must be viewed. At present they may augment the history and medical assessment in difficult diagnostic cases. They could also make a considerable contribution to psychiatric nosology.

3.

Critical comment on this statement brings forward discussion on the genetics and nosology of manic depressive illness. This has been a subject of increasing interest in the last 15 years. There is general agreement that manic depressive psychosis is inherited as research findings have shown concordance rates for relatives of 12 per cent, for dizygotic twins of 23 per cent and for monozygotic twins of 68 per cent. More recent Scandinavian research for concordance rates among monozygotic twins are lower. In recent years evidence has accumulated that unipolar and bipolar manic depressive illness may be inherited differently. It has been observed that from 50 concordant monozygotic pairs of twins from the total literature including both series and single case studies, 22 were observed to be unipolar concordant, 21 bipolar or manic concordant and seven unipolar/bipolar or manic concordant. These distributions are different to what would be expected if unipolar and bipolar disorders had an identical genetic background. It must be remembered however that observation on monozygotic twins does not clarify whether the genetic differences are due to specific or modifying genes. Information of this kind can only be derived from studies on dizygotic twins or on families where the modifying genes would be different. It has been observed from the literature that among 17 dizygotic twins concordant for manic depressive illness 10 were unipolar concordant, two bipolar concordant and five were unipolar/bipolar concordant pairs. These figures though small are not at variance with the assumption of distinct genetic entities. There are considerable difficulties however in drawing valid conclusions from these kinds of observations as environmental factors may modify or change the phenotype. Such environmental influences are well known in medicine. For example a patient with phenylketonurea put on a phenylalanine free diet at an early stage is less likely to develop the stigmata of phenylketonurea than a patient not on such a diet. At the time of birth monozygotic twins are not necessarily identical to each other as one of them may have been exposed to intrauterine disadvantage which might manifest itself by a change in phenotype. The question of whether unipolar depression is inherited differently to bipolar illness at present remains unresolved, but the trend of evidence is that they may be different, and that bipolar illness may have the greater heritability.

4.

Mixed affective states are those varieties of manic depressive disorder in which some of the features of mania and of depression are simultaneously co-existent. It is most commonly observed during the transition period from depression to mania or vice versa. They may be diagnosed as schizophrenic because of the variety of symptoms they present with. The simultaneous presentation of symptoms of depression and mania appears paradoxical and Kraepelin sought to explain it by describing six varieties of mixed affective states. Included among them are conditions he described as manic-stupor and depression with flight of ideas. Kraepelin's six conditions are not regarded as having nosological status.

Other efforts at explanation of these states include the occurrence of schizophrenia during the course of a manic depressive illness or the superimposition of hypomania upon depression. Conceptual models of a continuum and triangular type with mania, mixed states, depression and normality interposed at particular sites, have been proposed in an effort to understand the relationship of the affective phenomena to one another. There is no convincing explanation for this occurrence at present. Lithium is regarded as the treatment of choice in mixed affective states.

5.

Although there are many rating scales for depression there appears to be only one manic scale of promise. This was designed in 1971 by Beigel and his co-workers and has 26 items each one of which is rated on separate five point scales for frequency and intensity. It has a high inter-rater reliability and the advantage that it can be used by nursing staff who are in contact with the patient throughout the day. This scale is still relatively new but is likely to be of considerable help in quantifying manic behaviour and in delineating different types of manic depressive illness.

6.

This patient should be hospitalised in an acute psychiatric ward with close observation. Large doses of tranquillizers are indicated initially to control this patient's manic behaviour. As the patient is insightless, physically and verbally threatening, it is unlikely that he would accept oral medication so parenteral medication may be appropriate. Chlorpromazine 200 to 300 mgs intra-muscularly daily could be used. These dosages may have to be increased if the patient does not show signs of responding within 24 hours. As soon as feasible oral medication should be introduced and lithium should be prescribed dose adjusted by daily blood tests to achieve a blood concentration of 0.6 to 1.2 mmol/litre. Should the patient not respond to the above treatment a course of E.C.T. may be beneficial. After the acute phase of the illness has subsided the objective should be to maintain the patient on the treatment regime which has been successful in the past and ensure as far as possible that the patient complies with this by his frequent attendance at out-patients and a lithium clinic, and by enlisting the help of the relatives.

7.

There is evidence that rapid neuroleptization using parenteral agents results in faster remission of acute psychotic symptoms compared to oral pharmacotherapy. Neuroleptics are extensively metabolised by the liver and bioavailability after oral administration is decreased due to the hepatic first-pass effect and interahepatic circulation. For example the bioavailability of haloperidol given orally is reduced to 45 per cent to 60 per cent compared to parenteral administration and oral doses should be 1.4 or more times as large as perenteral doses to result in identical serum concentrations of the drug. Mean peak serum levels may take three hours or longer with oral medication whereas intra-muscular preparations may reach mean peak serum levels in 20 minutes. Some investigators however have suggested that giving neuroleptics intra-muscularly results in rapid sedation but not faster remission of psychotic symptoms than oral preparations, while others maintain that parenteral administration ameliorates core psychotic symptoms more quickly. As up to 50 per cent more neuroleptic may be required to attain comparable serum concentrations when oral rather than parenteral drug is given, there may be an increased likelihood of untoward effects from oral medication. Of course a distinct advantage of parenteral medication is that with acutely disturbed psychotic patients no other form of medication may be accepted by the patient.

Course and management

The patient responded satisfactorily to chlorpromazine 200 mg 6 hourly and lithium 800 mg nocte. The chlorpromazine was reduced to 100 mg t.d.s. after one week. After discharge the patient attended a lithium clinic regularly to monitor his serum lithium and observe his progress and he resumed his studies.

Further reading

Allen M G 1976 Twin studies of affective illness. Arch Gen Psychiat 33: 1476–1478

Beigel A, Murphy D Bunney W E 1971 The manic-state rating scale. Arch Gen Psychiat 25: 256–262

British Medical Journal 1981 Leading article — The new psychiatry. Brit Med J 283: 513–514

Menuck M Voineskos G 1981 Rapid parenteral treatment of acute psychosis. Comp Psychiat 22(4): 351–361

Trethowan W H 1981 Mixed affective states. Lundbeck Publication 1 (March)

CASE 6

A consultant psychiatrist is requested by a general practitioner to do a domiciliary visit to an elderly couple who are described as demented and unable to cope. There is one daughter who is married and living 25 miles away, has family commitments, and can only meet the parents twice weekly. The woman is aged 81 and the man is 79. They live in the ground floor flat of a large late Victorian house, the rest of which is unoccupied. There are four steps up to the door with a lounge, a dining room, a kitchen and scullery and cloakroom leading off a long rather dark hallway. There is also a lavatory on this ground floor, but the bathroom is situated on the first floor. The dining room functions as a bedroom. Although the house is clean there is a damp musty smell and the furniture is old. They receive meals on wheels daily, have a home help and a district nurse who comes twice weekly and they are known to the local social service area office. Shopping is done both by the daughter and the home help and the district nurse washes them regularly and bathes them at least once a week. It was arranged for the daughter to be present during the consultant's visit and she informed him that the mother has become increasingly confused over the previous 18 months and is becoming incontinent of urine and neglectful of her personal hygiene. She is inclined to wander out of the house, get lost, and on at least two occasions was brought back by the police in the early hours of the morning. The onset of her confusion was insidious and the daughter cannot relate it to any incident, illness or accident. There is no previous psychiatric history and no relevant medical history. At the interview the old lady is completely disorientated for time and place, knows nothing of current affairs nor can she name the present monarch or the prime minister. She cannot retain new information, but can name her daughter and her husband with difficulty. She does not know her address. In general remote memory, although embarrassed is better preserved than recent memory. She is not depressed and there is no clouding of consciousness. She is insightless on her condition and is incapable of giving a coherent history, she appears well physically. The daughter informs the consultant that the husband is well mentally and that if there is any confusion it is very mild. She continues that the husband's own problem is physical in that he has had increasing difficulty in walking since he fell and injured his back and broke two ribs nine months previously. He was treated in a casualty department for this, his ribs and his back were x-rayed and he was sent home. By holding on to the dresser and the back of a chair he can very hesitantly shuffle about three or four feet away from the chair he sits on. At interview he is generally lucid mentally, he knows the day of the week and the month but the date is inaccurate, and he relates this inaccuracy to not having a daily newspaper. He is reasonably well informed on current affairs, can name people prominent in public life and is familiar with current news items. He is not depressed, but experiences considerable anxiety about the wife's wandering and his inability to cope with it due to his relative immobility. The thought of locking the front door with a second key has occurred to him but he decided not to do this as he would take too long to open it for visitors and he and the wife could not readily gain exit in an emergency. There is no psychiatric history and no other relevant medical history. In recent months he has become increasingly housebound and cannot negotiate the front door steps and at times he says he feels isolated, lonely and bored, but he has never contemplated suicide.

Questions

1. What is your formulation on these patients?

2. Would you comment on the following statement — 'What is required for the ever increasing numbers of psychogeriatric patients is not so much a team of specialist physicians like in cardiology, but social supportive care such as can be as effectively provided by nurses, social workers and occupational therapists as by consultants!

3. What are the advantages and disadvantages associated with 'a psychogeriatric assessment unit'?

4. What effect may separation have on these patients?

5. What are the applications of the 'problem orientated medical record' in psychiatry?

6. How would you manage these patients?

7. Has the psychiatrist a role in a terminal care unit?

8. Briefly do you know of any methods of assessing life expectancy for patients with senile dementia?

Answers

Q1.

This elderly lady is probably suffering from moderately advanced senile dementia characterised by gross cognitive impairment, loss of insight and wandering. She represents a danger to herself from accident and exposure. The physically handicapped husband whose condition needs investigation is incapable of coping with her, especially with her wandering and she is a source of great anxiety to him. Even with considerable community support at present in the form of meals on wheels, home help, district nurse and visits from their daughter they are not coping. It would be ideal if they had a caring relative or friend living in the home with them. The wife is in need of psychiatric assessment and the husband of geriatric assessment, before long term planning is possible.

Q2.

Cardiology is very much a part of high technology medicine and psychogeriatric medicine is not. Nevertheless to provide an efficient effective service the psychogeriatrician needs a broad training with a knowledge of many aspects of health care and medicine as well as psychiatry and such broad knowledge is not to be found in members of paramedical staff, however dedicated. A good knowledge of geriatric medicine and of social medicine, neurology and neuropathology as they apply to the elderly is needed. He needs to have administrative ability and drive to lead a multi-disciplinary team and campaign for a fair share of resources for the elderly mentally infirm. He should also be familiar with and able to undertake epidemiological, biological and operational research. Unless the psychogeriatrician is able to do these things, he is not fully trained. To ameliorate, slow up and maybe some day reverse the 'irreversible' dementias is the central clinical challenge to the psychogeriatrician. This challenge can only be met by close co-operation between highly trained consultants in the clinical setting and medical scientists in the laboratory. There is no competition between cardiology and psychogeriatric medicine, indeed they should complement one another. A comprehensive psychogeriatric service is the cardiologists greatest asset in ensuring that an elderly psychogeriatric patient will not be inappropriately placed in one of his beds. It will also help to improve the quality of life for these elderly mentally infirm whose life span has been extended by high technology medicine.

Q3.

A psychogeriatric assessment unit has mainly a dual function. Firstly to investigate elderly patients with psychiatric illness particularly those with confusional states which may have a treatable organic basis. Secondly to assess what is the most appropriate form of placement, management and care. Of course this helps to ensure that patients are not misdiagnosed and misplaced, which could be distressing to the patient and costly to the health service. As the units are run jointly by the psychogeriatrician and the geriatrician this helps to ensure co-operation between the services and provides whole patient care. These units limit the period of assessment to four to six weeks and this helps to ensure that the patient does not loosen bonds with home, community and friends and does not becomes over dependant on the hospital. In practice the cost effectiveness of psychogeriatric assessment units have not been established. They may be costly to run as they require a high concentration of staff and many investigations are carried out. There is a strong tendency for patients to remain much longer than the four to six weeks planned, because there may be a shortage of outlet beds in the local psychiatric hospital and there may be a waiting list for residential accommodation. There is therefore a danger that the unit may take on some of the characteristics of a long stay psychogeriatric ward. Many of the functions of a psychogeriatric assessment unit could be carried out in an admission ward for the elderly in a psychiatric hospital which had access to a visiting consultant geriatrician and to facilities for physical investigations.

Q4.

It is likely that separation especially initially would have a deleterious effect on both partners. If the old lady is removed from the companionship of her husband and her familiar surroundings, it is likely that she will become more confused. Old confused people orientate themselves to some degree by reference to familiar persons and surroundings, and when in an unfamiliar environment they become anxious, and perplexed and they may exhibit such behaviour as wandering or aggression. It is always worthwhile allowing an elderly person time to settle into a new environment before concluding they are unsuitable for it because of initial problems they present. The old gentleman may experience feelings of guilt at separation from his wife or believe that he has abandoned her. He may also feel redundant and demoralised as the caring role he played towards his wife has now been removed from him and he may to some degree have become psychologically dependant on this caring role. The psychiatrist must be aware of these complications of separation, in formulating treatment programmes for a member of an elderly couple especially when they have lived together for many years.

Q5.

A correct psychiatric diagnosis is necessary for classification, it will also indicate prognosis and suggest useful treatment. However it frequently fails to fully explain or account for all the problems presented by a patient, assign priority to them and suggest solutions. The 'problem orientated medical record' (P.O.M.R.) does not represent an abolition of diagnosis but rather an expansion of it, and central to it is the compilation of a problem list. This list may go on the first page of a patient's case notes with the date when the problem was noted. The list is dynamic and solved problems are removed from it and maybe new ones added over a period. It is customary to subdivide the problem list into active or inactive and immediate attention of the therapeutic team is directed at the active problems. Inactive problems are those which cannot be readily solved within a reasonable period of time or are relatively insoluble. Frequently a problem will require further elucidation and in this case it is usual to indicate this by placing an arrow after the problem for example. In the present case for example for the female patient one could list problems of the active kind as-confusion, wandering, inadequate supervision and of the inactive kind as, no other tenant in the house apart from the elderly couple, and no bathroom on the ground floor. Further advantages of the P.O.M.R. is that even if the diagnosis is unclear or even false as may often be found in psychiatry, attention can still be directed at specific problems, the goals of the therapeutic team can be clearly stated and progress can be monitored. If a diagnosis becomes clear at a later date it can be introduced into the problem list as an active problem. The approach of the P.O.M.R. is consistent with the view that psychiatric illness is multifactorial in origin and frequently presents with many problems.

Q6.

In the first instance the wife should be admitted to a psychiatric hospital for further assessment and investigation of her confusion. If this confusion is due to a treatable condition such as an endocrine disorder, a depressive illness, a nutritional deficiency or a treatable cerebral condition then the objective should be to return her to her home eventually. If the confusion is due to senile or multi-infarct dementia, then she should be assessed to see if it were again possible for her to return home with further community support such as day hospital attendance. If there is an improvement in the husband's condition, especially his immobility then he may with help, manage to accept the wife back and control her wandering. Should home care not be possible then the patient might be acceptable for an elderly person's home, but her confusion, wandering and incontinence may militate against it. Permanent hospitalisation may be the last option. The husband should be referred for full geriatric assessment and the wife's long term management may be determined to a large degree by the husband's degree of improvement in his mobility.

Q7.

The psychiatrist can perform a very useful role in a terminal care unit. These units tend to have a much higher psychiatric referral rate than general hospitals. Nearly all these patients experience emotional distress of some kind especially during the early days of their stay. They may realise for the first time the seriousness of their illness. Reasons for referral may include depression, anxiety, abnormal behaviour patterns, communication problems between staff and patients, family and social problems and suicidal danger. Referred patients tend to be younger than the non-referred group, those under 50 years show more depression and anxiety, and mothers with children still at home are particularly at risk. Patients in a terminal care unit are usually on several drugs including narcotic analgesics, antidepressants, phenothiazines and butyrophenones for potentiation of analgesia or as antiemetics or muscle relaxants. The psychiatrist can successfully intervene in about 2/3 of referrals, by supportive psychotherapy, counselling and family therapy. The psychiatrist has a role in supporting staff who find care of the dying emotionally demanding and as an educator of staff so that someone will be able to respond to the psychological needs of a patient when a psychiatrist is not available.

Q8.

Studies have shown that males have poorer life expectancy than females, that patients who performed poorly on psychometric tests such as the Mental Test Score and the Digit Copying Test also had a poorer life expectancy than patients who did better. Impaired parietal lobe function also indicates poor prognosis. Computerised tomographic measures of ventricular size and cortical atrophy lack predictive value.

Course and management

The old lady was admitted to a psychiatric hospital for further assessment and was found to be suffering from advanced senile dementia and was considered incapable of living in the community and long term hospitalisation was required. It was considered unlikely that the elderly husband could cope with her increasing mental frailty. The old gentleman was admitted to a geriatric hospital for investigation and it was planned for him to live with his daughter on discharge.

Further reading

British Medical Journal 1981 Correspondence column. Brit Med J 283: 494–496

Copeland J R M, Kelleher M J, Barron G G, Cowan D W, Gourlay A J 1975 Evaluation of a psychogeriatric service. The distinction between psychogeriatric and geriatric patients. Brit J Psychiat 126: 21–29

Fry A 1978 Some aspects of the problem orientated medical record in general psychiatry. In: Gaind R N, Hudson B L (eds) Current themes in psychiatry I, Macmillan Press Ltd, London and Basingstoke.

Noguib M, Levy R 1982 Prediction of outcome in senile dementia: a computed tomographicy study. Brit J Psychiat 140: 263

Stedeford A, Bloch S 1979 The psychiatrist in the terminal care unit. Brit J Psychiat 135: 1–6

CASE 7

An 80-year-old retired lady is referred to outpatients by her general practitioner. She complains that 'I do things mechanically, I know everything around me is real but I cannot grasp its reality, and I feel unreal, when I look at myself in a mirror, it does not seem to be me'. Both parents died of natural causes many years ago, there were nine siblings in the family, she has very little contact with her siblings and describes them as not very close. Her early childhood years were unremarkable, and she did quite well at school, left at 14 and stayed at home until she reached the age of 21. She then got a job as a shop assistant in a tobacco shop chain and remained in that firm until she retired at the age of 65. She is heterosexual, had a few boy friends but never married and she does not smoke and drinks very little alcohol. She owns her one bed-roomed flat and has lived there for many years by herself. Up to her retirement from work she had a fairly good social life with many friends and visitors, but since her retirement her contact with her friends has diminished and she feels lonely. She describes herself as being 'always a sort of friendly person, liked travelling abroad a lot, but I could get moody at times'. Her past medical history is not relevant. 20 years previously she was admitted to hospital for the treatment of depression and says 'I recovered well with tablets' and has remained well since, she took tablets for two years after leaving hospital. She is quite sure that she felt depressed on that occasion and that there were no feelings of depersonalisation. Her present symptoms started about nine months previously and have followed a progressive course. She began to feel anxious, tense and depressed with considerable lack of energy and drive. Her sleep pattern was disturbed and she experienced difficulty in getting off to sleep and early morning waking. Soon she began to get feelings of depersonalisation and she eventually went to see her general practitioner and says 'when I thought I was going mad'. He prescribed tricyclic antidepressants which helped her during her previous psychiatric hospitalisation but on this occasion they appeared to be ineffective. She could not relate the onset of symptoms to any particular stress and the general practitioner finally referred her to psychiatric outpatients. On assessment she looks distressed, anxious and dispirited. She is clean and tidy in her attire, is co-operative and tries to be attentive but is pre-occupied with her depersonalisation symptoms and seems afraid that she is 'going mad'. She admits to feeling depressed, but denies suicidal intentions and there is no cognitive or perceptual disturbance and she appears to be well within the average intellectual range. She rarely leaves the flat and is isolated socially.

Questions

1. What is your diagnosis on this patient?

2. In which conditions may you encounter depersonalisation symptoms?

3. How do you distinguish between nihilistic delusions and depersonalisation feelings?

4. What do you know of the psychopathology of depersonalisation?

5. How would you treat this patient?

6. What adverse psychological effects may retirement produce?

7. Why do you think the antidepressants which helped her in her previous illness, appear to be unsuccessful in the treatment of her current illness?

8. Would you list drugs which may induce depression?

Answers

Q1.

This 80-year-old patient is probably suffering from an atypical phobic anxiety depersonalisation syndrome. This syndrome was first described in the 1950s and is characterised by diffuse anxiety and panic attacks. The panic attacks may be associated with both feelings of depersonalisation and derealization. Very frequently depressive symptoms with anorexia and weight loss (which the patient does not have) are components of the syndrome. The majority of sufferers are females in the 20 to 40-year-old group, and the syndrome is uncommon in a person of this patient's age. Electro con-vulsive therapy is reported as making the condition worse and anti-depressants are claimed to be usually effective.

Q2.
Depersonalization symptoms may be found in phobic anxiety states, temporal lobe epilepsy, temporal lobe migraine, depression, schizophrenia, L.S.D. intoxication, sleep deprivation, and in the hypnagogic state. They may be observed in people without a psychiatric or neurological disorder.

Q3.
Depersonalisation feelings do not qualify as delusions. The patient retains insight into his condition, realises it is strange and abnormal and may complain of it to the doctor. It may however be related to a disturbed perception of self and of the environment. Nihilistic delusions have the characteristics of true delusions in that they are false beliefs, are held with conviction, cannot be modified by an appeal to reason or logic that would be acceptable to people of the same religious or cultural background. Although patients suffering with depression or schizophrenia may present with both nihilistic delusions and depersonalisation, feelings of depersonalisation are more commonly associated with phobic anxiety states and depression and nihilistic delusions with schizophrenia. Depersonalisation symptoms may occur suddenly and remit spontaneously, and be relieved by social stimulation.

Q4.
There is no definitive view on the psychopathology of depersonalisation. In psychoanalytical writings depersonalisation is claimed to serve a protective function for the organism and is a defence against aggressive feelings and overwhelming anxiety. It has also been described as a 'preformed functional response of the brain', and represents one of a limited set pattern of responses by which the organism responds to innumerable agents real or imagined which may harm it. It has been compared to an exaggerated or inappropriate nociceptive withdrawal reflex. Another hypothesis is that it represents a disorder of recognition of personal identity or more precisely that there is a dissociation between the recognition of personal identity (which may be retained) and the recognition that this identity belongs to the self. It is of interest that some people report that depersonalisation occasionally but not exclusively occurred when they looked in a mirror, although they could identify their image, it did not appear to belong to them. This disorder of recognition has also been claimed to be of importance in the etiology of agoraphobia and paradoxically in feelings of déjà-vu, when the

whole of current experience becomes imbued with a sense of belonging, normally only accorded to the body.

Q5.

It would be worthwhile treating this patient with other antidepressants as an outpatient. One of the newer generations of antidepressants with minimal cardiotoxic effects would be appropriate. Over a period of three or four weeks she may respond to these so that no further psychiatric intervention apart from periodic attendance at outpatients for a few months would be needed. If she failed to respond to one type of antidepressant than another type should be tried and attendance at a day centre or a day hospital may be indicated so that she would have social stimulation.

Q6.

Retirement may have considerable adverse psychological effects comprised mainly of depression, anxiety and social isolation, especially on those who live alone and are unprepared for retirement. It may induce a sense of uselessness or of not being wanted or of not belonging and this is bad for the individual's morale and precipitates depression in vulnerable individuals. There is also a loss of companionship and of the social activities frequently found among working groups. Worrying about financial matters and difficulties in meeting financial commitments, when inflation threatens to overtake pensions and savings instills anxiety. The individual forcefully realises that he has indeed entered the declining years and the threat of physical and mental frailty and death is more real. Those individuals who are members of a family group, and have prepared for retirement by developing outside interests and hobbies and work for firms who take an interest in their ex-employees by providing clubs and social activies for them are obviously an advantaged group. The unemployed and the redundant will also experience some of the stresses of the retired.

Q7.

While it is good practice to re-prescribe antidepressant drugs which have helped an individual with a particular illness in the past, quite frequently it is found that they may be ineffective. The reasons for these observations are unclear as members of the two major groups of antidepressants, that is the tricyclic and mono amine oxidase groups, have in general similar biochemical actions to other members of this group. It is important to remember however that a depressive illness presenting at one stage of life may not be identical to one preceding it at another stage and that the etiology of depression is multifactorial. Also over a 20-year period or less the environmental stresses on an individual could change considerably as could his ability to cope and deal with them. Time-induced biological changes within the individual, could also change in a subtle or gross manner the effectiveness and influence of drugs on him. However, it is good practice to try another antidepressant or member of a different group of antidepressants on an individual who is unresponsive to one.

Q8.

It is difficult to say with certainty in the individual case that a specific drug caused depression. This is because depression is frequently multifactorial in origin and the drug may be just one of these potential factors. Nevertheless experience has shown that some drugs are more likely than others to induce depression. Included among these are hypotensives, such as reserpine, clonidine, methyldopa and probably some beta adrenoceptor blocking drugs such as inderal and pindolol. Corticosteriods such as cortisone and prednisone may also do so. The incidence of depression is higher among those on oral contraceptives than among controls. Although bouts of depression are common in Parkinson's disease, nevertheless it is most probable that levodopa ('larodopa', 'brocadopa') can also cause depression. Appetite suppressants especially fenfluramine (ponderax) may also cause depression. Neuroleptic drugs such as fluphenazine enanthate (moditen) and fluphenazine decanoate (modecate) have also come under scrutiny as inducers of depression, but it is by no means clear that they do so, as depressive disturbance quite frequently is found in association with schizophrenia. Other drugs which have also been incriminated include griseofulvin (fulcin) digoxin (lanoxin) and indomethacin (indocid).

Course and management

The patient was treated as an outpatient with one of the newer tricyclic antidepressants. She attended a psychogeriatric day hospital thrice weekly. After approximately one month she had improved considerably and though feelings of depersonalisation persisted the patient was not upset by them.

Further reading

Fogin L 1981 Depression and the recession. Med News (11 June): 23–24

Myers D H, Grant G 1972 A study of depersonalisation in students. Brit J Psychiat 121: 59–65

Roth M 1959 The phobic anxiety depersonalisation syndrome. Proc Roy Soc Med 52: 587

Salvage J 1981 The jobless mind. Nursing Times (24 June): 1103

Sim M, Gordon E B 1976 Basic psychiatry, 3rd edn, Churchill Livingstone. Edinburgh, London, New York, p 194–195

Tyrer P J 1981 Drug-induced depression. Prescribers Journal 21 (August): 237–242

CASE 8

She is a 74-year-old woman, who believes her husband is plotting against her and is having affairs with young girls. She is very verbally aggressive to the husband, and has been admitted to hospital at the request of her general practitioner under Section 25 of the Mental Health Act 1959. She came from a working class background, had one sister and two brothers; both parents died of natural causes and her siblings were killed during the second war. There is no history of psychiatric illness in the family background or of childhood neurotic traits in her early years. She attended school until she was 14 and was a reasonably good student. She is heterosexual, had the menarche at 16 and married a bank clerk at the age of 29, the marriage being described as 'very good in the past'. There are two daughters, aged 40 and 43, married with families of their own. Premorbidly she was described as domineering and extroverted, with many friends, sociable, liked to mix with others and was interested in dancing. Her previous medical history is irrelevant, but she had been thoroughly investigated previously at a general hospital for 'forgetfulness' and diagnosed as suffering with cerebral atrophy. Her history of aggression to the husband and of believing him to be unfaithful is of 18 months duration, but her history of forgetfulness is of two and a half years duration. Over the same period she had to be supervised in looking after the domestic duties and the husband does the shopping as she is unable to cope. She is not incontinent. On assessment she appears to be well preserved physically, is pleasant and co-operative during the interview and readily admits to having a poor memory. She is disorientated for time and place and with difficulty can name prominent people in public life. Her concentration is poor, she is not hallucinated and she describes herself as feeling 'sad' because of the way she believes her husband is behaving, but she is not depressed. She is unable to retain new information and her remote memory is better preserved than her recent memory. Her belief that the husband is unfaithful is intense and she says 'he wants to get my money, my stocks and shares, and get rid of me so that he can carry on with young girls'. It was ascertained from the daughters that there was no truth in the patient's allegations about the husband and he was indeed quite caring.

Questions

1. What is the differential diagnosis?

2. Apart from disturbance of memory what other disturbances are noted in senile dementia?

3. In which psychiatric conditions may you find morbid jealousy?

4. Is violent behaviour associated with morbid jealousy?

5. Have cerebral vasodilators a role in the treatment of this patient?

6. How would you manage this patient?

7. Very briefly what do you understand by the term 'late paraphrenia'?

Answers

Q1.

It is most likely that this woman's persecutory delusion has arisen from a misinterpretation of events because of her underlying cerebral atrophy. It is also possible that she is suffering with paraphrenia along with the cerebral atrophy, but her pre-morbid personality was not of the paranoid type. Paranoid delusions are also frequently found, of course, in schizophrenia and depressive illness but this woman is not schizophrenic and she is 'sad' rather than depressed. She is not taking any drugs which would induce a paranoid psychosis.

Q2.

There is deterioration in personality, social deterioration and behavioural disturbances. There is coarsening of the finer, more attractive aspects of personality, the social graces become less apparent, the patient may become sexually uninhibited and indecent exposure may take place. There is a loss of interest in appearance and the standard of personal hygiene falls, lability of mood with stereotypy of speech and conduct may become apparent. Gross behavioural disturbances such as aggression and violent behaviour may be exhibited. Neurological disturbances with signs of aphasia dyspraxia or pyramidal disorders may develop depending on the areas of brain tissue involved. Epileptiform attacks occasionally occur and the patient eventually becomes bed-ridden and incontinent. The duration of survial in general is about three to four years.

Q3.
Morbid jealousy may be a symptom of alcoholism, schizophrenia, personality disorder, drug abuse and depression.

Q4.
Serious violence may be associated with morbid jealousy, especially in a young couple when one member believes the other is unfaithful. Separation of the couple may be justified to prevent violence, but this may not be sufficient as a second partner may be a potential victim.

Q5.
A role is claimed by some pharmaceutical companies for cerebral vasodilators in the treatment of dementias, particularly in the early stages of vascular dementia. The consensus of current medical opinion is that there is no scientific or observable clinical justification for such a claim.

Q6.
As this woman's cerebral atrophy is likely to be progressive, management will have to be on a long term basis. It would be desirable in the first instance to plan discharge home after treatment with tranquillisers in moderate dosage which may remove some of the intensity from the delusions. The husband may need considerable support, as he is elderly. A home help and meals on wheels may be indicated and visits to outpatients and home visits by a community psychiatric nurse may encourage the husband to continue caring. Attendance at a psychogeriatric day hospital is of considerable help to a patient like this and gives a caring relative considerable relief. In the long term when mental and physical disability becomes marked the question of long term hospitalisation will have to be discussed.

Q7.
There is considerable discussion on the existence of paraphrenia as a distinct clinical entity since the word was first introduced in the 1950's. The debate has centred mainly on its relationship to paranoid schizophrenia and whether it could be regarded as a late form of schizophrenia. Late paraphrenia is a term used with reference to certain paranoid states of the elderly, not related to organic or drug induced causes but considered to be a modified form of schizophrenia. It comes on late in life, is most commonly seen in elderly

women living alone and is characterised by prominent paranoid delusions with or without hallucinations.

Course and management

The intensity of the patient's delusions decreased after a period of hospitalisation. She was treated with a moderate dose of thioridazine, attended an occupational therapy department for diversional therapy and was discharged to the care of the husband. She attends a psychogeriatric day hospital three days weekly and will be admitted at intervals to give holiday relief to the husband. The consensus of opinion was that she is suffering from a paranoid delusional state in the setting of moderately advanced senile dementia. The prognosis is poor and it is likely that she will need admission again in the near future.

Further reading

Bergmann K, Foster E M, Justice A W, Matthews V 1978 Management of the demented elderly patient in the community. Brit J Psychiat 132: 441–449

1979 Vasodilators in senile dementia. Brit Med J: 511–512

Grahame P S 1982 Late paraphrenia. Brit J Hosp Med 27(5): 522–528

Jolly D J, Arie T 1978 Organisation of psychogeriatric services. Brit J Psychiat 132: 1–11

Mowat R R 1966 Morbid jealousy and murder, Tavistock Publications, London

CASE 9

A 29-year-old man is referred from outpatients for admission. He complains that someone is using black magic and voodoo against him, of hearing voices which comment on his behaviour and shout and swear at him. He is distressed by this and is contemplating suicide. Both parents, who have a business, are alive and well, and there are two younger sisters and a brother. There is no family history of psychiatric illness. The patient was born in Jamaica, when his mother was 15 years old, and he was reared mainly by his maternal grandmother. His parents emigrated to England and he was united with them when he was 15. His childhood was not very happy due mainly to the fact that he did not mix well with his brother and sisters, he used to hide in corners and was very backward at school. Temper tantrums were frequent during his childhood and he remembers spending hours in front of the mirror combing his hair. He is described by a relative as always 'a bit difficult, shy and retiring, unable to concentrate, and poor at school and had many admissions to psychiatric hospitals'. He has never been able to work or hold down a job. There is no relevant past medical history and his first admission to a psychiatric hospital was 13 years ago when he was described as suffering with schizophrenia and subnormality. He has had six admissions to hospital since then at intervals varying from 18 months to two and a half years and the diagnosis has always remained the same. While in hospital he has been treated with phenothiazines and E.C.T. There is no history of alcohol or drug abuse. He has made two suicidal attempts in the past, when he was depressed because the voices were particularly derogatory and abusive, on one occasion he jumped into the river and was pulled out by river police and on another occasion he drank paint. At present he complains that the voices are particularly marked and very abusive. He feels depressed because of this and has contemplated suicide. On examination he appears quiet and rather withdrawn, there is no spontaneity of thought or movement, and he sits rather listless with an expressionless face. He smiles and laughs occasionally for no obvious reason, and at times appears to be preoccupied as if he were listening. He is obviously auditorily hallucinated and deluded — believing that the voices are being transmitted from Jamaica. He also feels that he is not fully in control of himself but is controlled by voodoo and black magic. He feels others can read his thoughts. Considerable difficulty is experienced when he tries to do simple calculations or name the days of the week backwards and he can only read in a slow childish fashion. Physical examination is negative. His present medication is fluphenazine decanoate 100 mg IM weekly and trifluoperazine hydrochloride 5 mg t.d.s.

Questions

1. What are Schneider's first rank symptoms of schizophrenia?

2. How many are present in this patient?

3. What are the advantages and disadvantages in the use of Schneider's first rank symptoms diagnostically?

4. How does subnormality influence the presentation of schizophrenia?

5. What do you understand by the Present State Examination (P.S.E.)?

6. How would you treat this patient?

Answers

Q1.
These are symptoms described by Kurt Schneider, a German psychiatrist, as being of first rank importance in the diagnosis of schizophrenia, each symptom is diagnostic in the absence of brain disease or intoxication. Briefly they consist of:-

a. Auditory hallucinations which may take the form of voices commenting on the patient's actions, repeating the patient's thoughts out loud or two or more voices discussing the patient or referring to him in the third person.

b. The experience of thoughts being put into the patient's head (thought insertion) or being withdrawn (thought withdrawal).

c. That the patient's thoughts are made known to others (thought broadcasting).

d. The feeling by the patient that his acts and feelings are controlled by an outside agency and he is just a robot.

e. That he is receiving bodily sensations from an outside agency passively or against his wishes.

f. The presence of delusional perception, that is a genuine perception which would be regarded as commonplace by a normal person, but of special significance to the schizophrenic giving rise to a fully fledged delusion.

Q2.

This patient has thought broadcasting auditory hallucinations commenting on his behaviour, his behaviour is under the control of an outside agency — black magic or voodoo. His delusion about voices being transmitted from Jamaica is not a delusional perception of first rank significance, but rather an attempt to rationalise his auditory hallucinations, which would not be regarded as genuine perceptions.

Q3.

The main advantage of Schneider's first rank symptoms is that they are easier to recognise and define than other criteria, for example, Bleuler's fundamental symptoms. In international studies of schizophrenia, Schneider's symptoms have proved highly discriminating. The main criticism of the symptoms are that up to 30 per cent of patients who would be regarded by psychiatrists as having schizophrenia do not have the symptoms when the diagnosis is being made and 20 per cent of chronic schizophrenics have never been known to have the symptoms. It is important to remember, however, that there is probably no symptom absolutely pathognomonic for a specific condition in medicine or psychiatry.

Q4.

The clinical picture of schizophrenia may be considerably altered by the presence of subnormality. Hallucinations may be gross, and of a primitive nature depending on the degree of subnormality and these may be presented in a childish monotonous fashion. Poverty of thought and what could be described as silly behaviour is prominent. Stereotypies and mannerisms are also frequently observed. It is important to distinguish between signs and symptoms which may be commonly observed in subnormality especially in the mentally and physically subnormal such as certain motor abnormalities and stereotypies. It is also important to remember that there is a high prevalence of low grade mental deficiency among schizophrenics.

Q5.

The Present State Examination is a method of interviewing patients which can be used by the psychiatrist after he has had a period of training in the technique. Its use by trained personnel results in high inter-rater reliability. The ratings are processed by a computer programme named CATEGO and this gives a standarised diagnostic grouping, which nullifies the diagnostic prejudices or bias of the interviewer. It is a flexible interview instrument in that there are certain probe questions which indicate the most likely fruitful line of questioning to be followed. It is very good for the diagnosis of schizophrenia but less accurate for organic psychoses and neuroses. It has had widespread use in international studies comparing diagnoses and in biochemical and pharmacological research on groups of psychiatric patients where accuracy of diagnosis is imperative.

Q6.
Due to the acuteness of his symptoms and his suicidal thoughts it is advisable to admit him to hospital. Treatment with large doses of intra-muscular anti-psychotic preparations should continue and these may be supplemented with oral phenothiazines. He should be observed in the ward setting until his symptoms become less acute and his suicidal ideas depart, but diversional occupational therapy should continue. If he fails to show signs of improvements over a period of two weeks, then because of the depressive element in his presentation and the obvious distress he is in, a course of E.C.T. should be considered. When improved he should attend a central occupational therapy unit and on discharge he should be followed up by the community psychiatric nurse who will give him his injection, report on his mental condition, give support to the family and ensure he attends a day hospital. Support for the family is imperative for his survival in the community and he could be admitted to hospital at intervals to give them holiday relief.

Course and management

On admission he was found to have a full scale I.Q. of 60 and a reading age of eight years. He responded to a combination of fluphenazine decanoate I.M. and chlorpromazine orally. He maintained his improvement and was discharged after four weeks to attend a day hospital daily. The hallucinations remained but he was not disturbed by them and he was not suicidal. Long term follow up with admissions for relapse and holiday relief is envisaged.

Further reading

Davis J M 1976 Recent developments in the drug treatment of schizophrenia. Amer J Psychiat 133: 208–214

Kendell R E 1972 Schizophrenia — the remedy for diagnostic confusion. Brit J Hosp Med October 82: 383

Koehler K 1979 The first rank symptoms of schizophrenia, questions concerning clinical boundaries. Brit J Psychiat 134: 236–248

Mann A, Murray R 1979 Measurement in psychiatry. In: Hill, Murray, Thorley (eds) Essentials of postgraduate psychiatry, Academic Press, ch. 4, p. 89

Reid A H 1972 Psychoses in adult mental deficiency. Schizophrenia and paranoid psychosis. Brit J Psychiat 120: 213–218

CASE 10

A 25-year-old girl is admitted to hospital under compulsory order by her general practitioner because she was 'behaving in a bizarre fashion, was extremely active, very loquacious and expressed over inflated ideas of her own importance'. Both parents are alive, she lives with them and is the second of three children. The father is a scientific instrument salesman and the mother is a secretary. The mother had two admissions for treatment of depression. The patient claims to have had a good relationship with both parents, there were no childhood neurotic traits. She liked school and was usually near the top of the class at examination time. She is a bright intelligent heterosexual girl of aesthenic build, interested in biology and travel. Her previous medical history is irrelevant but she has had two previous admissions to psychiatric hospitals, the first about two years previously and the last about 14 months ago, on both occasions being diagnosed as suffering with hypomania. After her last hypomanic bout she suffered with mild depression. For about one month prior to admission she appeared to be deteriorating mentally, she refused to continue with lithium tablets as she believed she did not need them and thinks she is 'becoming toxic'. She has been hyperactive, seems to need little sleep and has been very talkative and argumentative. She has expressed many impractical ideas and flits very quickly from one topic of conversation to another. Many of her ideas have been rather grandiose and flamboyant. At interview she is a tall girl who believes there is nothing abnormal about her and that she should not be in hospital. It is difficult to assess her mentally and she is argumentative and unco-operative. Her pressure of ideas and speech is obvious and she exhibits flight of ideas. She is full of self-confidence, easily distracted and has grandiose plans for the future. She thinks she is pregnant even though she wears a coil and her periods are not overdue. She is very critical of psychiatrists and reveals her views on the qualities of a good psychiatrist and says, 'If I stay in this hospital long enough I will wind up as a very good psychiatrist not a patient'. She is not hallucinated and although she expresses grandiose ideas she does not appear to be deluded. She is well physically and there is no history of drug abuse.

Questions

1. What is the diagnosis?

2. What do you know of the genetics of manic depressive psychosis?

3. Do you know of any psychoanalytical views on hypomania?

4. How does the prophylactic effect of lithium on hypomania compare with its effect on bipolar depression?

5. What are the contra indications to lithium and what precautions must one take in prescribing it?

6. What are your views on possible therapeutic mechanisms of action of lithium?

7. How would you treat this patient?

Answers

Q1.

It is nearly certain on the basis of her history and her presentation that the patient is suffering from hypomania.

Q2.

There appears to be a very mixed genetic factor in its etiology. The relatives of affected individuals have an increased risk (circa 12 per cent) and monozygotic twins show a much higher concordance rate (68 per cent) than dizygotic twins (23 per cent). The mode of transmission is unclear; both monogenic and polygenic methods have been proposed. It has also been proposed that unipolar and bipolar affective illnesses are inherited by different mechanisms and that predisposition may be by means of an X linked dominant gene.

Q3.

A classical psychoanalytical view on mania was that it resulted from a relaxation of the control of the super ego over the ego with the result that many repressed wishes rise to consciousness and that there is an accompanying mood which could be described as the mood appropriate to wish fulfilment. Mania has also been regarded as a defence mechanism against depression and unhappiness.

Q4.

The prophylactic effect of lithium on mania and hypomania appears to be well established by double blind placebo controlled studies. Most psychiatrists now also regard it as having a prophylactic effect on bipolar depression but this is not so well established. There is some evidence that it may be effective also in preventing recurrent unipolar depression.

Q5.

It is important to ensure that renal function is normal and that cardiac insufficiency, Addison's disease or frank hypothyroidism are absent. During pregnancy there is an increased incidence of cardio vascular malformations in 'lithium babies'. It should be ascertained that diet and fluid intake are normal. Any drugs affecting electrolyte balance (e.g. diuretics, appetite suppressants, steroids) may alter lithium excretion and should be avoided. Other psychotropic drugs should be used at lower dosage as their effects may be potentiated by lithium, of particular importance is the concurrent use of haloperidol and flupenthixol. There have been rare isolated reports of possible interactions between lithium and diazepam (hypothermia) methyldopa, propranolol and tetracyclines. Lithium and haloperidol in conjunction is contra indicated.

Q6.

The method of action of lithium remains to be established. It has been suggested that it influences the amount of sodium available for transfer across the cell membrane. It has also been suggested that it may have an effect on brain amine metabolism, hormonal imbalance and may function as an adenyl cyclase inhibitor, and so reduce the level of cyclic adenosine monophosphate. Research has tended to try and understand its method of action in the context of what is already known of the biochemistry of bipolar depression.

Q7.

In patient treatment is necessary and compulsory hospitalisation is required for observation as the patient is unwilling to remain informally, also the patient would be unreliable at present in taking medication if she were unsupervised. A combination of lithium with a neuroleptic drug should control the symptoms. Serum lithium levels should be performed as a guide to dosage, and in most patients the optimum concentration lies between 0.7 and 1.3 M.Eq/1 in blood samples drawn 12 hours after the last intake of lithium. When improvement occurs trial leave at home and eventual discharge can be planned. The neuroleptic may be reduced or omitted but it is important to explain to the patient the need to continue Lithium treatment for the long term, even though she may feel well, as discontinuation may lead to relapse. Attendance at an outpatient clinic for observation and frequent estimations of serum lithium is necessary. Decrease in frequency of serum estimations is possible with increase in the period that the patient has remained well. If toxic effects appear, lithium treatment should cease, a serum lithium should be performed and the patient should be encouraged to drink plenty of fluid.

Course and management

The patient improved considerably on chlorpromazine 150 mg t.d.s. and lithium 800 mg nocte over a period of three weeks. She absconded from the hospital before expiry of Section 25 but continued with medication and attended outpatients regularly. She returned to work, has continued with lithium and remains remarkably improved. The prognosis is reasonably good provided she continues with treatment.

Further reading

Mendels J 1971 Relationship between depression and mania. Lancet 1: 34

Price J 1968 The genetics of depressive disorder. In: Coppen A, Walk A (eds) Recent developments in affective disorders, Headley Bros, Ashford, Kent p. 35–54

Quitkin F, Rifkin A, Klein D F 1976 Prophylaxis of affective disorders. Current state of knowledge. Arch Gen Psychiat 33: 337–341

Schou M, Amdisen A, Baastrup P C 1971 The practical management of lithium treatment. Brit J Hosp Med July 3: 5

CASE 11

A 70-year-old man living alone is referred to hospital by his general practitioner because he is depressed and confused. Both parents died of natural causes, two brothers are alive and well and there is one sister who is a chronic psychiatric inpatient. His wife died of heart failure about seven months previously and apparently the marriage was a happy one. From information from the daughter who accompanies him it appears he had a difficult childhood because of poor financial circumstances in the family. The father died quite young during the great flu epidemic in 1919. The patient worked at unskilled jobs. He describes himself as 'easy going and sociable', but the daughter describes him as 'stubborn, quick tempered and moody'. One year previously he was found on investigation to have positive V.D.R.L. and T.P.H.A. tests when he was brought by his family to hospital because of forgetfulness and depression. He was referred to a venereal disease clinic for further investigation and treatment where he received a course of procaine penicillin injections. He did not keep follow up appointments. There is no previous psychiatric history. The daughter says that over the previous six months the patient has become withdrawn and depressed, he has neglected his personal hygiene, has become increasingly forgetful and disorientated, his appetite has deteriorated, he is sleeping poorly tending to wake in the early morning and is making increasing demands on her and her sister, both of whom have their own family commitments. At interview he is depressed and apathetic, showing little interest in the interview, and is dishevelled in appearance. He is disorientated for time but not place and has difficulty in naming people prominent in public life. He can retain new information with difficulty. He is not suicidal, there are no delusions or hallucinations evident. On physical examination an ejection systolic murmur is audible along the left sternal margin and neurologically there is diffuse increased muscular tone and loss of vibration sense in both lower limbs. Psychological testing concludes there is organic brain damage and also severe depression.

Questions

1. What is the differential diagnosis?

2. What is pseudo dementia?

3. Describe the more common neurological and psychiatric aspects of general paralysis of the insane.

4. What role has the clinical psychologist to play in the assessment and care of the organically confused elderly patient?

5. How would you manage this case?

6. What precautions must one take in prescribing tricyclic anti-depressants for a patient in this age group?

Answers

Q1.

There are a few diagnostic and inter-related contributory possibilities to be considered in this case. It is clear from the history and from observation and psychological assessment that there is a distinct depressive element in his presentation. His positive serology and neurological signs and confusion suggests that general paralysis of the insane must also be considered although this is now an extremely rare condition and most unlikely in isolation to be the main cause of his symptoms. His confusion may possibly be explicable in the setting of his depression as depressed elderly can present with confusion (pseudo dementia). Probably the best procedure in the first instance is to regard this as a unipolar depressive illness in an elderly person on the basis a precipitating factor (the death of the wife), the depressed mood and the disturbance in sleep and appetite. Immediate re-referral to a veneral disease clinic is, of course, necessary.

Q2.

In old people unipolar depression may present more prominently with a picture of dementia than with affective disturbance. There may be neglect of personal hygiene and deterioration in habits even to the degree that there may be incontinence of urine. It may be differentiated from true dementia by the more acute onset, and by the observation that the cognitive impairment is not as pronounced and by the presence of morbid and self critical remarks and ruminations. There may also be a family history of depression, with presentations in this fashion. The response to antidepressants and/or E.C.T. may be marked with resolution in depression and confusion. Few psychiatrists, however, have difficulty in distinguishing true dementia from pseudo dementia and of course depression and dementia may co-exist.

Q3.

The Argyll Robertson phenomenon is not common but incomplete forms may be commonly observed. Signs of pyramidal system disturbance are common such as increased tendon jerks and extensor plantar responses. There may be loss of control of bladder and rectum with incontinence, and sexual impotence may be present. Generalised convulsions are common and death may occur following a fit. When an element of tabes dorsalis is present tendon jerks may be absent. Tremor of the tongue, the limbs and the lips may be present, speech is hesitant, indistinct and irregular. Mentally, dementia is the most constant and overriding feature of the condition. All other features are determined by the degree of neurological damage, the patient's previous personality and his experiences. The expansive grandiose presentation is not as common as is generally believed. Atypical presentations with depressive or hyperkinetic features may be observed and presentations with paranoid, catatonic and hysterical features have been described. Expansive delusions and statements are observed if the patient's previous personality tended towards euphoria and grandiosity or if he was over ambitious or unrealistic about the goals he wished to achieve.

Q4.

The role of the clinical psychologist in assessment and care is considerable and should be viewed in the context of the multidisciplinary therapeutic team. It is necessary to view results from tests in conjunction with other tests and re-testing is necessary over a period of time to monitor progress or deterioration. The experienced psychologist can test for type and degree of cerebral impairment and give an indication of rehabilitative possibilities. The Wechsler Deterioration Indices are very widely used to measure organic impairment. A discrepancy of greater than twenty points between verbal and performance abilities on the W.A.I.S. gives a statistically significant indication of organic impairment as verbal abilities are more resistant to deterioration than performance abilities. Other useful tests in diagnosing organic confusional states are the Modified Word Learning Test, and the Paired Associate Learning Test. Perceptual and motor perceptual tests used to diagnose organic disorders include the Minnesota Percepto-Diagnostic Test and the Graham-Kendall Memory for Design Tests. The psychologist's role is one of on-going assessment and advice rather than of a 'one off' assessment shortly after admission.

Q5.

It would probably be advisable to admit this patient to hospital, because of his history of recent positive serology, for psychological and psychiatric assessment and for treatment of his depression. Re-referral to the venereology department is necessary and treatment of his depression with tricyclic antidepressants, preferably with those reported to have less cardiac dysrhythmic effects is indicated and the medication could be given at night to promote a more normal sleep pattern. Psychometric testing to ascertain the degree of organic impairment and/or depression should be performed. If unresponsive to antidepressants over a period of three or four weeks a different antidepressant could be tried and/or E.C.T. considered. It may be observed that with improvement in his affective state he may present a much more lucid picture mentally and depending on his degree of residual impairment which should be assessed again after improvement in his depression, long term management plans hopefully outside the hospital should be formulated.

Q6.

Before prescribing tricyclic antidepressants for the elderly patient one should ensure that there is no disorder of cardiac rhythm history of recent cardiac infarction, prostatic hypertrophy or closed angle glaucoma. Patients should be warned of the anticholinergic effects which may cause dryness of the mouth, blurred vision and constipation. The newer tricyclics or tetracyclics may sometimes be considered more appropriate.

Course and management

The patient was admitted and responded well to amitriptyline 75 mg nocte. He completed a second course of procaine penicillin. When his depression subsided he was much more lucid and independent but there was still some cognitive impairment. He was discharged to a warden supervised flatlet and attended outpatients at intervals and an occupational therapy unit. Consensus opinion favoured regarding this man as suffering from endogenous depression in the setting of a mild to moderately advanced dementia in which syphilitic infection of the nervous system may have been a contributing factor. The prognosis for the foreseeable future may be reasonable with appropriate supervision.

Further reading

Dewhurst K 1969 The neurosyphilitic psychosis today. Brit J Psychiat 115: 31–39

Forrest A D, Affleck J W, Zealley A K (eds) 1978 Tricyclic drugs. In: Companion to psychiatric studies, Churchill Livingstone, Edinburgh, London, New York, p 543

Post F 1972 The management and nature of depressive illness in late life: a follow through study. Brit J Psychiat 121: 393–404

Whitehead A 1973 Verbal learning and memory in elderly depressives. Brit J Psychiat 123: 203–208

CASE 12

A 17-year-old girl is referred to psychiatric outpatients from the casualty department of a general hospital where she had been treated for an overdose of barbiturates and alcohol. She is of no fixed abode and has been living rough in central London for about two years. She says she is 'accepted as part of the scenery there now'. She is the third of four children, her parents separated when she was about two and she and her siblings were placed in care. She remembers seeing her mother on one occasion four years previously and remembers the father visiting the home to see her at irregular intervals. She describes him as alcoholic, illiterate and aggressive. She tried to stab him on one occasion. She occasionally has contact with the youngest sibling but does not have any details of the two older ones. After being reared and educated in a series of four children's homes she left the last one at the age of 15. At school she was regarded as bright and she claims that her teachers told her she could do 'O' or 'A' levels if she applied herself. Her interests are in art and English and she claims to be a warm person who would 'like to have a job helping people'. She finds difficulty however in establishing enduring relationships with others. After leaving the home she worked at various jobs for short periods, such as Wimpy bars, Hot Dog stands and 'tried prostitution for a while', but she has not worked at any job for more than a few months. She is heterosexual, had one boy friend who died in an accident six months previously. In the past she suffered 'with fits' when she was withdrawn from barbiturates but is otherwise well physically. There have been four previous admissions to psychiatric hospitals because of suicidal attempts in the form of wrist slashing or overdosing. While in hospital she broke windows and physically attacked other patients. Her abuse of drugs started when she was 11, she claims, 'I took speed at 11, smoked cannabis and took barbiturates at 13'. She claims to 'need something every day' and says, 'If I haven't got a drug I'll take alcohol', but denies that she is dependent on any particular drug. At the age of 13 she was sent to a Remand Home because of her general bad behaviour, possession of drugs and overdosing. She appeared in Court at the age of 17 after having been 'picked up in Piccadilly with methadone, speed and cannabis and got a conditional discharge'. For the past weeks she says she felt life was not worth living, felt very depressed and 'took an overdose of tuinal and alcohol and decided to collapse somewhere other than Leicester Square so they wouldn't find me'. She was unconscious for 24 hours after admission to hospital and still feels life is not worth living. She relates her depression intimately to her deplorable life style, and expresses a wish to move out of London, settle down and get a job. At interview she looks depressed and gives the impression of still being suicidal. There is no cognitive or perceptual disturbance and she appears to be of good average intelligence with no evidence of brain damage subsequent to repeated periods of unconsciousness after overdoses. There are no obvious withdrawal effects from drugs apparent. She expresses a wish for help and is willing to come into hospital informally.

Questions

1. What is your formulation on this patient?

2. Briefly discuss the concept of 'the psychopathic personality'.

3. What are the principles of the therapeutic community as applied to the treatment of personality disorder?

4. Which developmental and psychodynamic views of the etiology of psychopathy do you know of?

5. How would you treat this patient and what is the prognosis?

6. What do you know of psychiatric disorder in children in long term residential care?

7. What is your concept of an adolescent psychiatric unit?

Answers

Q1.

This 17-year-old girl is suffering with a depressive suicidal state and has a poor personality with psychopathic traits. Her personality deficit has been largely contributed to by her disturbed and deprived early childhood, having especially been deprived of contact with her mother in her early years and having been reared in institutions. Part of her problem at present is that she is rootless, homeless and without a stable adult figure to whom she can relate. Her depression is probably reactive to her difficult life situation and her willingness to be admitted to hospital may reflect her desire to escape from this.

Although she has abused both alcohol and drugs she does not appear to be physically dependent on them. Her personality development has been severely impeded and she is incapable of relating maturely to individuals or society, so treatment will have to extend over a number of years and success will depend mainly on her motivation and desire to improve.

Q2.
The concept of the psychopathic personality is elusive and there is not at present general agreement on its existence as a distinct psychiatric condition. Nevertheless the weight of opinion seems to be coming round to the view that it is a separate entity, a form of mental disorder separate from psychosis, neurosis and mental subnormality, though it may present in conjunction or in association with these conditions. Confusion has arisen mainly because of the overlap of psychopathic and criminal behaviour and the difficulty in assessing to what degree an individual is simply 'bad' rather than 'mad' and also because patients with neurotic or psychotic conditions or subnormality of intelligence can develop psychopathic behaviour patterns. In general terms the psychopath is an individual who exhibits irresponsible or aggressive behaviour out of keeping with the sociocultural norms in which he lives, who has poor insight into his condition, who does not learn by his mistakes, who makes society and/or himself suffer as a result of his actions and has little capacity for feeling remorse or for reform.

Q3.
The principle of the therapeutic community is to provide a social learning situation, for an individual (especially the psychopathic person) so that he may develop new ways of social interaction and examine why his current behaviour patterns are socially unacceptable. The individual is encouraged to partake in the management and running of the community. This instils a sense of responsibility and a feeling that he has something worthwhile to contribute. Antisocial or maladaptive behaviour is discussed by groups of residents so the motivated individual develops insight into his abnormal pattern of behaviour. The group formulates its rules and discipline and group and individual responsibility is encouraged. The liberal and democratic method of the therapeutic community is thought to be conducive to the development of maturity and responsibility in individuals for whom the professional authority in a large institution would be deleterious. Poor motivation on the part of the individual would limit its effectiveness, and the ability to adopt

a responsible role in a therapeutic community setting does not guarantee the ability to do so in the general community. Also achievement of maturity may take many years in patients with psychopathic personalities. Overall however, the therapeutic community approach to treatment of psychopathic personalities is a very worthwhile endeavour to manage a very intractable condition.

Q4.

Developmentally parental deprivation in the very early years of life is thought to be conducive to the condition. Parental attitudes especially of rejection have also been considered of importance as have erratic standards of parental behaviour. Psychoanalytically, the psychopathic personality is immature in emotional and personality development and considered to be fixated at a proto phallic level and there is a poorly developed super ego. This fixation results in impulsivity, lack of remorse, guilt or restraint. Ego strength is weak in contrast to an overwhelming id.

Q5.

In the first instance this girl should be admitted to hospital for observation as she is probably still suicidal. The intensity and nature of her depression should be assessed and it may well respond to manipulation of the various stresses which have effected her rather than to antidepressants. It should become apparent after two or three weeks whether the willingness to come to hospital merely reflected a temporary wish to escape from an intolerable life style outside or also a genuine and ongoing wish to change. If she is unmotivated then it is likely she will leave hospital after the immediate crises have subsided and return to her old pattern of behaviour. If she is willing to remain in hospital then many possibilities for treatment can be considered, including referral to a therapeutic community or adolescent unit for admission or advice, attendance for group or individual psychotherapy, aimed at helping her to relate in a mature responsible manner to individuals and society. If she improved she could then be referred to an after care hostel and attend a career training or industrial therapy unit. It is likely that she would need ongoing supervision and guidance for many years. A mature sympathetic adult such as a social worker or community psychiatric nurse and preferably a female to whom she could turn for help and advice, would have a key role to play in the long term management of this patient, she would be a surrogate parent yet have professional insight and skill. Success will ultimately depend largely on the patient's motivation. The prognosis for the foreseeable future is poor and she may kill herself intentionally or inadvertently.

Q6.

There is evidence that a large percentage of children in long term residential care show signs of psychiatric disorders. At any one time there are approximately 95 000 children in the care of local authorities in England and Wales and of course children in long stay establishments only form part of these. The most common disorders noted in 'long term' children are of neurotic and anti social types. It is also a cause of concern that at follow up over a period of years there is persistence of these disorders. It has been suggested that persistence of these disorders particularly of anti social behaviour is due to a vicious circle of unacceptable behaviour and adult rejection.

Q7.

Adolescent units differ considerably in their admission policies, treatment environments and their duration and method of follow up. Adolescents with anxiety depression or phobic disorders, those with anti social behaviour or sexual problems and those with difficulties in relating to peers or adults are considered for treatment. Psychotic and subnormal patients are in general not considered suitable for treatment. Motivated youngsters benefit most and the unit works in close liaison with the family. Many adolescents will return to their parents at weekends and a therapeutic contract or plan is formulated between the staff, the patient and the family. There is a high staff patient ratio and each patient may be allocated a particular member of staff as a counsellor. The aim of the unit may be to modify destructive ways of behaving by restricting 'acting out', and by providing frequent opportunities for 'talking out' problems. There is daily group therapy as well as groups in art therapy and psychodrama. Improvement in up to 80 per cent of neurotic disorders and 50 per cent of conduct disorders has been claimed, but recurrence of the main presenting symptom in a milder form is common.

Course and management

The patient's depression subsided quickly without medication within a week of admission to hospital. Plans were made for her to receive individual supportive psychotherapy twice weekly and attend an assessment unit with a view to receiving sheltered employment while remaining as an inpatient. She absconded after four weeks took an overdose of tablets and was readmitted from a casualty department after one week. She absconded again after five weeks and did not seek readmission.

Further reading

Lewis A 1974 Psychopathic personality — a most elusive category. Psychol Med 4: 133–140

Thorley A, Stern R 1979 Neurosis and personality disorder. In: Hill, Murray, Thorley, Essentials of postgraduate psychiatry, Academic Press, London, P 231–237

Wells P G, Morris A, Jones R M, Allen D J 1978 An adolescent unit assessed: a consensus survey. Brit J Psychiat 132: 300–308

Whitely J S 1970 The psychopath and his treatment. Brit J Hosp Med 3: 263
Wolfkind S, Renton G 1979 Psychiatric disorders in children in long term residential care. A follow up study. Brit J Psychiat 135: 129–135

CASE 13

A 45-year-old man with a history of heavy alcohol consumption over a period of 20 years is admitted to hospital after a domiciliary consultation. He is restless, agitated and sweating and has been without alcohol for the previous two to three days. Both his parents are dead and he is the fourth of nine children; his mother was treated in a psychiatric hospital for depression on one occasion and one of his sisters committed suicide at the age of 19. There is no other psychiatric history in the family background. He claims to have had a reasonably happy childhood and there were no obvious childhood neurotic traits. He was a moderately good student, left school at 16 and did semi-skilled clerical work for many years until he was sacked for absenteeism and because the quality of his work had deteriorated and he was abusive and aggressive to his employers. In recent years he has worked mostly at labouring jobs. Normally he is a warm friendly personality but can be difficult and argumentative when under the influence of alcohol. His social life has centred on pubs and clubs where alcohol is readily available. He married at 25 but was divorced six years later due mainly to his drinking behaviour; there were no children. At present he lives with his nephew. He has been drinking since the age of 19 and has had two previous psychiatric admissions, one three years previously and the other in the preceding year both for the treatment of delirium tremens. He denies a criminal record but he has been 'barred from certain pubs and warned by the police for being drunk and disorderly'. Normally he drinks beer, will drink up to eight or nine pints daily and will also drink whisky if, he can afford it. His appetite has been indifferent or poor for many years. His tolerance for alcohol has decreased in recent years and he cannot now drink as much as he used to. If alcohol is not available he becomes agitated and tremulous. He has not had any alcohol for about two days, and says he awoke on the kitchen floor after experiencing what he 'thought was a fit'. He also experiences what he describes as 'black outs' and is worried by these. At interview he appears to be in good nutritional state, he is obviously restless and tremulous, but there is no evidence of psychotic features or cognitive disturbance, apart from worry about 'fits and black outs'. There is no evidence of depression. On physical examination his liver is 4 cm below the costal margin, is tender and smooth, his pulse rate is 110 and his blood pressure is 160/90 and all his reflexes are brisk. There is no jaundice evident. He admits to having an alcohol related problem and states that he intends to abstain.

Questions

1. What is your formulation on this case?

2. What do you know of the aetiology of alcoholism?

3. How would you explain this patient's 'fits' and 'blackouts'?

4. Which psychiatric disorders may be associated with alcoholism?

5. What contribution does alcohol abuse and dependence make to criminality?

6. How would you treat this patient?

Answers

Q1.

This man is suffering from chronic alcoholism as a result of which he has suffered physical and possibly mental damage. At present he appears to be in an incipient phase of delirium tremens due to his abstinence from alcohol for two to three days. He appears to have some insight into his problems and expresses an intention to abstain. His lack of adequate family support, his single status and the fact that his social outlet has always centred on visits to the pub, will militate against his plans for abstinence or compliance with a treatment programme. Hospitalisation for treatment of his physical condition and further assessment is necessary.

Q2.

The aetiology of alcoholism is complex, multifactorial and inter-actionary and the relative importance of causative factors may vary among individuals. Alcoholism is two to three times more prevalent among the parents and siblings of alcoholics than among the general population, and this suggests, but does not prove, a constitutional or genetic predisposition. Twin studies also suggest a genetic pre-disposition. Environmental influences may also be important. Bio-chemical theories on differences between alcoholics and non-alcoholics exist but so far no consistent fundamental biochemical abnormality has been described, although much interest has focussed on the enzyme alcohol dehydrogenase. Attempts to describe an alcoholism prone personality as lacking in confidence, self destructive, latently homosexual, immature and orally fixated have not met with general success, although individual alcoholics may exhibit one or more of these personality traits. Psychologists have studied alcoholism in the context of learning theory and conditioning. Alcoholism has high rates in certain races and cultures such as the French and Irish, and low rates among Jews, possibly due to cultural and social factors. Certain occupations are also associated with high rates for alcoholism, such as those of bar tenders, waiters, journalists, members of the armed forces and commercial travellers. Alcohol is often freely and cheaply available to these groups. The higher incidence of alcoholism among men than women is decreasing due to social changes.

Q3.

The patient's 'fits' and 'blackouts' could probably be explained in the context of alcohol associated neurological disorders. Convulsions are common among alcoholics and may occur during acute intoxication or withdrawal or they may be due directly to cerebral damage. In individuals prone to epilepsy alcohol may precipitate an attack. 'Fits' and 'blackouts' may also be seen in alcoholic degeneration of the corpus callosum (Marchiafava's disease) and in alcoholic dementia.

Q4.

The best known psychiatric disorder is the confusional state associated with delirium tremens. This confusion may be associated with delusions and hallucinations of a vivid nature, and is usually associated with marked physical disturbance especially of the autonomic system. Tranquillisers have helped to reduce the severity of the condition. Morbid jealousy is also associated with alcoholism, the alcoholic may accuse the spouse of being unfaithful and this may be accompanied by violence and threats of violence. It is thought to arise from increasing impotence on the part of the alcoholic and a refusal by the partner to partake in sexual activity while the spouse is drunk. A state of auditory hallucinations of a derogatory nature occurring in clear consciousness may be observed in alcoholism and is described as alcoholic hallucinosis. Alcoholics may also experience lapses of memory or periods of amnesia which are commonly described as 'black outs'. In long standing alcoholics deterioration in personality and intellect has been described, the finer points of the personality are blunted and he becomes more demanding, self-centred, dependent, and exhibits emotional outbursts. There is a well established association between alcoholism and such conditions as Wernicke's encephalopathy and Korsakoff's syndrome.

Q5.

There is a close relationship of alcohol abuse and dependence to culpable negligence, violence and criminality in general. A high percentage of motorists involved in or killed in road accidents have high blood alcohol levels. Many violent incidents are to be observed either in public houses or in their environs after closing hours. Alcohol intoxication leads to impulsive behaviour and argumentative conversation which may result in physical assault or homicide. Alcoholics have many times the suicide rate of controls and 40 to 50 per cent of short term prisoners have a drinking problem and/or were drunk at the time of committing their offence.

Q6.

This patient should be admitted for treatment of his physical condition, rehydration, chlormethiazole and intravenous vitamins should control his subacute delerious state. When he has recovered, liver function tests should indicate the degree of liver damage present and thorough neurological and psychological assessment is necessary. His long term management depends to a large degree on his motivation. He could be referred to an alcohol treatment unit for admission but he may not be accepted as he may be regarded as lacking motivation and of particularly poor prognosis. Alternatively he could be treated within the hospital setting with group psychotherapy and attendance at Alcoholics Anonymous meetings. After discharge from hospital the patient could attend a day hospital and continue his association with Alcoholics Anonymous. Disulfiram may be helpful in reinforcing the patient's intention to abstain. A club or social outlet should be provided for the patient to reduce the temptation to return again to the pub and to fill the vacuum in his social life. Outpatient follow up for the long term is necessary.

Course and management

The patient was admitted to hospital and was treated with diazepam 10 mg t.d.s. for one week and he was physically much improved after about three days. He expressed an intention to abstain from alcohol and he was treated with Disulfiram tabs. one mane preceded by a Disulfiram controlled reaction and discharged from hospital after ten days. He was introduced to the local branch of Alcoholics

Anonymous and attends outpatients and an expatients' club. Prognosis for this type of alcoholic patient is not good due to lack of family support and poor motivation and also because he has no social outlet apart from visits to the pub.

Further reading

Costello R 1975 Alcoholism treatment and evaluation I and II. Int J Add 10: 251–275, 857–867

Cutting J 1982 Neuropsychiatric complications of alcoholism. Brit J Hosp Med 27(4): 335–342

Davies P 1979 Motivation, responsibility and sickness in the psychiatric treatment of alcoholism. Brit J Psychiat 134: 449–458

Edwards G, Heasman C, Peto J 1971 Drinking problems among prisoners. Psychol Med 1: 388–399

Murray R 1979 Alcoholism (psychological disabilities). In: Hill, Murray, Thorley (eds) Essentials of postgraduate psychiatry. Academic Press, London, New York, p 325–326

Pearce J M S 1977 Neurological aspects of alcoholism. Brit J Hosp Med 18: 132–142

Sillanpaa M 1982 Treatment of alcohol withdrawal symptoms. Brit J Hosp Med 27(4): 343–350

CASE 14

A 28-year-old woman is referred to a psychiatric outpatients department by her general practitioner because she is agitated, depressed, and feels tense and aggressive and the symptoms appear to be related in time to her premenstrual period. The father is dead; there are three other siblings in the family and she is the second eldest. There is no family history of psychiatric illness, but the patient describes her mother as 'neurotic'. She claims to have had a generally unhappy childhood as they had to move frequently because her father worked as a semi-skilled worker and had difficulty in holding down jobs. This upset her school attendance considerably. Her parents divorced when she was 15. She claims to have been fairly good at school and left at 16. There were no childhood neurotic traits evident. She was 'very attached' to the father, but never got on well with the mother. After leaving school she worked mostly at clerical jobs, with an insurance company, a timber company, and a shipping agent. She had her menarche at the age of twelve and she has her periods regularly. They last about five days and occur every 28 days. She has a boyfriend of four years duration by whom she has two children aged three and one and they live together as common law husband and wife and in general their relationship is satisfactory. She was treated for depression as an outpatient after a termination of pregnancy ten years previously and was also treated as an inpatient in a psychiatric hospital five years later after a suicidal attempt with an overdose of tablets while she was depressed. She has been described as a histrionic immature personality in previous reports, and appears to be of good intelligence. Over the last four or five years she has noticed a periodicity to her symptoms of anxiety, restlessness, and tension, which appear to be related to the week before the onset of menstruation. She becomes extremely short tempered with the boyfriend and the children and has been tempted on two or three occasions to push her daughter down the stairs because she could not move out of her path quickly. She was, however, never violent to the child. She also complains that she feels bloated and is convinced that she has considerable fluid retention during this time and that this fluid interferes with her vision because it accumulates behind her contact lenses. Headache is also present. During this time she feels angry rather than depressed 'and will jump at anyone who talks to me'. The onset of menstruation appears to relieve the symptoms to some degree. At interview she is in the postmenstrual phase, is without psychiatric symptomatology and her mood and affect are appropriate and normal.

Questions

1. What is your formulation on this case?

2. What is your view of the premenstrual tension syndrome as a distinct clinical entity?

3. Which biological theories of premenstrual tension have you heard of?

4. Would this patient's personality described as histrionic and immature and her psychiatric history of depression be of importance in the genesis of her symptoms?

5. How would you treat this patient?

6. Is there a relationship between psychiatric morbidity and gynaecological problems?

Answers

Q1.
This woman appears to be suffering from a syndrome commonly described as premenstrual tension characterised by emotional disturbance, irritability and a tendency to be abrupt, short tempered and aggressive, which is periodic in onset and is related to a period varying from 2–10 days before the onset of menstruation. It may also be characterised by a subjective feeling of being bloated, or of retaining fluid. It is relieved by the onset of menstruation. Its relationship to menstruation suggests that it is related to hormonal imbalance occurring during the premenstrual period.

Q2.
Although considerable discussion still occurs on the existence of the premenstrual tension syndrome, there is general agreement that although the majority of menstruating women have some symptoms of premenstrual tension there are those who experience particularly severe mental and behavioural abnormalities related to the premenstrual period. Doubt on its existence as a clinical entity arose because to investigators the symptoms did not appear with such regularity as to suggest a possible association with the premenstrual period and because of a suggestion that women who complained of premen-

strual symptoms had an increased tendency due to attention seeking traits in their personality, to complain of tension and irritability at other times as well. The fact that no consistent hormonal, biochemical or psychological explanation for these symptoms has been found also tended to cast doubt on its existence. There are now many studies showing a relationship to the premenstrual period of suicidal thoughts, and of emergency psychiatric outpatient appointments, and the symptoms have been described in differing cultural and ethnic groups.

Q3.

Biological theories of the premenstrual tension syndrome have centred mainly on the absolute, or relative circulating levels of the hormones, oestrogen, progesterone and luteinising hormone. High levels of circulating oestrogen and/or a relative deficiency of progestational hormones to oppose the action of oestrogens has been postulated as causative. An allergic sensitivity to endogenous sex hormones has also been suggested as operative. It has also been suggested that the normal monoamine oxidase activity changes during the cycle may be related to changing levels of progesterone, which in turn may be of importance in causing symptoms. Attention has also focussed on premenstrual water retention, but this does not appear to be the cause, nor have studies on pelvic congestion and fibrosis, or glucose metabolism provided an answer. In brief no consistent biological or hormonal basis for premenstrual tension has been found.

Q4.

The close relationship in time of this woman's symptoms to her premenstrual period and the relief of her symptoms by the onset of menstruation suggests that her symptoms are predominantly due to premenstrual tension. Nevertheless it is likely that a histrionic, immature personality would draw more attention to her symptoms and exaggerate them. It has been suggested that personalities who experience unsatisfactory childhood relationships in their family and who are unable to cope with day to day problems have some correlation with premenstrual tension. There is also an association between premenstrual affective symptoms and clinically significant affective disorder and neuroticism as described by the Maudesley Personality Inventory and this woman has a history of depression.

Q5.

At present there is no uniformly effective treatment regime. Different types of treatment have been tried with varying degrees of success claimed, but no consistently successful treatment programme has evolved. Forms of treatment which have been tried include radium thereapy to the ovaries, use of progesterone and of oestrogens to reduce hypothesised imbalances, also synthetic progestational agents such as oral contraceptives have been tried. Theories suggesting that salt, and water retention are etiological factors have resulted in the use of water restriction and diuretics, and vitamin thereapy has also been tried. Some of the foregoing treatments however, have produced results showing no significant differences with the use of placebo. This patient could be referred for hormonal assay to establish if there is any related hormonal imbalance. She could also have a therapeutic trial of a range of hormonal tablets which may include the contraceptive pill, to establish which, if any, give her greatest relief. As this woman has a history of depression and there appears to be an association between premenstrual affective symptoms and clinical affective disorder a trial of treatment with an antidepressant and supportive psychotherapy may be indicated.

Q6.

There is considerable psychiatric morbidity reported in associatin with gynaecological problems. It has been reproted that about 10 per cent of women attending gynaecological outpatients are psychiatrically unwell and half of them are of menopausal age. High scores for neuroticism have been noted in women in gynaecological outpatients, especially those with menorrhagia. Hysterectomy is over represented in surgical procedures assocaited with post operative psychoses. This may be due to an excess of depressed women complaining of symptoms which result in eventual hysterectomy. Women attending gynaecological outpatients are more likely than the general population to have had previous contact with psychiatric services. Depression and anxiety and irritability are common conditions observed. Premenstrual tension has of course received considerable gynaecological and psychiatric scrutiny.

Course and management

The patient refused a simple trial of hormonal treatment and was referred for a full hormonal assay but she did not keep appointments or return to Outpatients. The prognosis for the foreseeable future is unclear.

Further reading

Balbinger B C 1977 Psychiatric morbidity and the menopause: a survey of a gynaecological outpatient clinic. Brit J Psychiat 131: 83–89

Sampson G A 1979 Premenstrual syndrome: a double blind controled trial of progesterone and placebo. Brit J Psychiat 135: 209–215

Sampson G A, Jenner F A 1977 Studies of daily recordings from the Moos menstrual distress questionnaire. Brit J Psychiat 130: 265–271

Sampson G A, Prescott P 1981 The assessment of the symptoms of premenstrual syndrome and their response to therapy. Brit J Psychiat 138: 399–405

Tonks C M 1968 Premenstrual tension. Brit J Hosp Med 1: 383–387

Wetzel R D, Reich T, McClure J M, Wald J A 1975 Premenstrual affective syndrome and affective disorder. Brit J Psychiat 127: 219–221

CASE 15

A 54-year-old woman is referred by her general practitioner because she is depressed, feels she is very evil, is possessed by the devil and controlled by him and hears voices repeating her thoughts. She is not suicidal and says that it would not help her to escape the 'devil enemy'. Her father is dead but her mother is still alive and living with her. She describes the mother as extremely overprotective and she makes all the patient's decisions. There was one sister who died of natural causes six years previously and there is no psychiatric history in the family. She had a happy healthy childhood and was academically mediocre at school. There were no childhood neurotic traits. She left school at 16 and worked at the Ministry of Defence as a semi-skilled worker for 30 years. She is not working at present. There was a relationship of 12 years duration with her future husband before they married when she was aged 51. She used to see him one evening per week and this was chosen by the mother and after the marriage the mother tried to ensure that the same arrangement would continue. Previous to her first psychiatric illness three years ago she claims she was a warm friendly person with a small close circle of friends. She denies that she was over religious, but says she was always very dependent on the mother. She was interested in reading and television. Her medical history is irrelevant and she had her first admission to psychiatric hospital two years previously, when she was diagnosed as suffering with 'depression and religious delusions' and treated with antidepressants and E.C.T. Since then she has been admitted twice to hospital with a similar presentation and has been treated with chlorpromazine and trifluoperazine. Her last admission was six months previously. She relates the onset of her psychiatric problem to shortly after her marriage when she and her mother moved in to live with her husband, who already had his mother and a single brother living with him. There was considerable friction in the house as the patient's mother tried to dominate and control the relationship between the patient and the husband and pressurized the patient to move out of the home which she did six months after entering. Shortly after that she had her first psychiatric illness. Her delusions have persisted since her first presentation two years previously but she is more depressed and upset by them in the last two to three weeks. She relates her depression to the unpleasant delusions. She is not quite sure whether she was depressed by the difficult home situation before the onset of the delusions. In the past she claims to have heard the voice of the devil and seen him 'with a head like that of a goat'. She recently

heard her thoughts spoken out loud. At present she is not hallucinated. Her sleep and appetite are undisturbed and she is uniformly depressed throughout the day. There is no cognitive defect.
She is of good average intelligence and she does not take unprescribed drugs. Her present medication comprises chlorpromazine
and trifluoperazine in moderate dosage. She appears depressed and
agitated and is deluded, believing she is possessed by the devil.

Questions

1. What is the differential diagnosis?

2. What is your concept of schizoaffective psychosis?

3. Discuss the term "schizophrenogenic mother"?

4. What do you know of the relationship of 'life events' to the onset
   of psychiatric illness?

5. What do you know of personal construct theory and schizophrenia?

6. How would you treat this patient?

7. Have you heard of the word 'oneirophrenia'?

Answers

Q1.

The diagnoses that need to be considered in this case are as follows:- Firstly that she is suffering from schizophrenia, and has clear
cut symptoms of this such as delusions that she is controlled by the
devil. She has passivity feelings and recent hallucinations in the form
of her thoughts spoken aloud and has exhibited schizophrenic first
rank symptoms in the past. Depression should also be considered.
She admits to feeling depressed. The adverse home situation may
have precipitated it and the content of her delusions could be seen
in the setting of a depressive illness. She could also be described
as suffering with a schizoaffective illness with features suggestive
both of schizophrenia and depression. The possibility that this
woman's symptoms are basically a hysterical response to escape from

an overpowering mother and an intolerable home situation cannot be ignored, although there is no evidence that she is a hysterical personality type or has any history of hysteria, and one must be very careful in diagnosing hysteria for the first time in a patient of this age.

Q2.
There is considerable discussion on whether patients with schizophrenic-like symptoms in the setting of a marked depressive component, with precipitating factors, with rather quick remissions and a relatively good prognosis without permanent defect should be included in the schizophrenic category. The term schizoaffective is inclusive but is regarded as a 'hedging of bets'. Some regard these individuals, on the basis of the frequency of depression in the family background, as having a variant of depressive illness, while others regard them as occupying a position on a spectrum between schizophrenia and depression. Others still regard them as representing a separate group of cycloid psychoses. Included in the term schizoaffective in the ninth Revision of the International Classification of Diseases are cycloid schizophrenia, mixed schizophrenia and affective psychoses, and schizophreniform psychosis affective type.

Q3.
The schizophrenogenic mother is a term coined to describe certain characteristic abnormalities which are thought to exist in the mothers of schizophrenic patients and which are conducive to the development of schizophrenia in the children. It is thought that these mothers are overprotective of the children and assume an intrusive and dominating role in their lives. It has not been shown however that these maternal traits have not developed in response to the behaviour of a child who is already abnormal. There does appear to be general consensus at present that mothers of schizophrenic patients differ from controls in being over concerned.

Q4.
It has been shown that many psychiatric patients, especially schizophrenics and depressives experience more disturbing life-events in the weeks or months preceding the onset of their illness than do controls. For schizophrenic patients these occur approximately three or four weeks before relapse, but for depressives they may occur many months before and be a source of on-going worry and anxiety. The disturbing life-events may take the form of occupational, family, or financial crises, bereavements or socially disturbing occur-

rences. The precise role of life-events in precipitating the illness, or the degree to which they accelerate its onset remains to be decided. It is thought that for schizophrenics life-events just trigger off the illness, which would have occurred later in their absence, but these events may be causative for a large percentage of depressives.

Q5.

The personal construct theory of George Kelly proposes that each individual has his own set of constructs, that is, a mental process whereby he relates, interprets and makes meaningful his everyday experiences, e.g. if an individual's concept of physical robustness is related to his concept of aggression, then all physically robust people may be regarded as aggressive. It is hypothesised that schizophrenics have loosely connected constructs which result in difficulty in interpreting the environment meaningfully. This hypothesis would support the 'double bind' theory whereby abnormal family communications disrupt and prevent a child from developing a healthy construct system by placing him in impossible situations, not amenable to rational solutions and so may lead to thought disorder. However tests for schizophrenic thought disorder based on this theory have not a high correlation with other indices of schizophrenia.

Q6.

The patient should be admitted to hospital for further assessment and observation. The relationship between mother and daughter should be investigated and on the assumption that if it is psychologically damaging to the daughter the possibility of doing family therapy with both of them of an explanatory and supportive type should be pursued. It is unlikely that the mother will change her attitude to the patient, but methods of coping with the mother's attitude and of seeking help before a crisis develops should be explored. With previous hospitalisations the patient improved quickly and it is likely that she will do so again. Chlorpromazine in moderate dosage should continue and if the the depression does not subside with hospitalisation then a tricyclic antidepressant could be prescribed. It is unlikely that ECT will be necessary. After discharge attendance at a day hospital a few days weekly for therapy and observation would be advisable. Efforts to reunite the patient with the husband in their own accommodation should be made.

Q7.

Oneirophrenia is a state characterised by multiple scenic hallucinations in which the patient loses all contact with his surroundings.

The condition may last for weeks. It is described in the American literature, as closely related to schizophrenia and is thought to be due to a confluence of schizophrenic and affective genes. The term 'oneiroid states' is sometimes used.

Course and management

Concensus opinion favoured regarding this patient as suffering with schizoaffective psychosis. The mother refused to be involved in family therapy. The patient improved very quickly after hospitalisation and she was treated with chlorpromazine 50 mg t.d.s. and was discharged to attend a day hospital. The immediate prognosis is not good, but the long term prognosis may be better. Schizoaffective patients in general have a better prognosis than frank schizophrenic patients.

Further reading

Bannister D 1962 The nature and measurement of schizophrenic thought disorder. J Ment Sci 108: 825–842

Brown G W, Birley J L T, Wing J H 1972 Influence of family life on the course of schizophrenic disorders: a replication. Brit J Psychiat 121: 241–258

Leff J P, Hirsch S R, Rohde P, Gaind R N, Stevens B C 1973 Life events and maintenance therapy in schizophrenic relapse. Brit J Psychiat 123: 659–660

Procci W R 1976 Schizoaffective psychosis: fact or fiction. Arch Gen Psychiat 33: 1167–1178

Vaughn C, Leff J P 1976 The influence of family and social factors on the course of psychiatric illness. Brit J Psychiat 129: 125–137

CASE 16

A 72-year-old man is referred to a psychiatric hospital for admission from the casualty department of a general hospital where he had been treated for an overdose of nitrazepam taken with the intention of killing himself. The patient lives alone. He never married. The father was killed in the first world war and the mother committed suicide at the age of 34 while depressed. Apart from the mother's illness there is no history of psychiatric illness in the family. There is one sister alive and well. As far as the patient knows he was a full term normal baby and there were no childhood neurotic traits. He appeared to be a reasonably good student and left school at the age of 14. He changed jobs frequently for the first three years after leaving school and finally he trained as a carpenter and had completed his training by the age of 20. Shortly afterwards he joined the Royal Airforce and remained there until he was 37 years old and since then he worked as a carpenter up to the age of 65 when he retired. He is heterosexual and had two relationships with women, but his plans for marriage were disturbed by the second world war. He describes himself as conscientious, but shy and retiring, especially towards women. He has few friends and he does not make friends easily. Occasionally he visits the pub where he drinks moderately and he smokes about 20 cigarettes daily. Apart from watching television, reading, and the occasional visit to the pub he has few pastimes. His past medical history is irrelevant and there is no previous psychiatric history. The living accommodation, comprising a self-contained flat, is satisfactory. At interview the patient is quite obviously depressed and remarks 'Oh' why didn't they let me die? Why didn't I succeed? I don't want to be a burden or live till 'I'm 90'. The patient was found semi-conscious, lying on the floor, by the police after a neighbour informed them that she had not noticed him moving around and could not get a response when she knocked on the door. The patient relates the onset of his problems to when he was charged and convicted for stealing a tin of salmon from a supermarket three months previously and was given a conditional discharge. Since then he has felt that the police and the neighbours are watching him, though he thinks he could have been depressed even before he was charged, maybe for up to a period of a year. He has been depressed uniformly throughout the day. His sleep is good, but he takes one or two nitrazepam tablets to get off to sleep and his appetite is poor. He has lost interest in his daily activities, is lacking in energy and cannot mix with people. He feels very guilty, that he has wasted his life, and he worries excessively, especially about financial matters and says 'I think my supplementary benefit will stop if the D.H.S.S. know that I have saved £400.' On examination he is a suicidally depressed, tall, grey haired man, and is extremely apologetic about 'causing trouble to everybody'. He is very agitated and anxious. There is no cognitive disturbance or evidence of hallucinations, but he thinks the police and the neighbours are watching him. He appears to be of average intelligence and is in good general physical health.

Questions

1. What type of depression is this patient suffering from?

2. How do you assess the likelihood of this patient committing suicide?

3. Do you know of possible relationships between early death of this patient's parents and his sucidal attempt?

4. Do you know if shop lifting is associated with certain psychiatric conditions or has psychiatric connotations?

5. Has E.C.T. a place in the treatment of this patient?

6. Do you know of psychological theories on the mode of action of E.C.T.?

7. What is the treatment and long term management of this patient?

8. Apart from anorexia nervosa, what other disorders of eating are found in psychiatric practice?

Answers

Q1.

This patient is suffering with atypical depression, that is with features suggestive of endogenous and reactive types, but the features are mainly suggestive of the endogenous type. The fact that he has what could be described as a good personality which up to recently has coped with stress and worry would suggest an endogenous type of illness. Poor appetite, loss of interest in his hobbies and activities and the lack of energy and drive and feelings of unworthiness and guilt would support the diagnosis of this type of depression. Also elderly endogenously depressed patients frequently present with marked agitation. The fact that the patient largely relates the onset of his depression to his conviction for shop lifting suggests that this was the stress to which he responded with a reactive type of depression and difficulty in getting off to sleep is claimed to be a prominent feature of reactive depression. It is important to keep in mind that a psychological trauma such as a conviction for shop lifting can also trigger off an endogenous type of illness or exacerbate a pre-existent illness and this patient admits to feeling unwell even before his conviction.

Q2.

There is no accurate method of assessing the likelihood of suicide in this man but no threat can be ignored. In general it is fairly well established that the incidence of suicide is higher in large industrial communities, among the elderly, more among men than women especially those who live alone, among ex-patients and alcoholics, among single people and among those without religious affiliations. In particular, in assessing the individual risk a positive history of previous suicidal attempts, especially those of a genuinely serious nature, people with depression and a positive family history of suicide and the presence of a readily available method of killing themselves, such as access to drugs or firearms, all increase the danger.

Q3.

Some studies have shown a higher rate of early parental death, especially maternal death among depressed patients, than among other psychiatric patients and of course, depression is the illness most intimately associated with suicide. Research has also suggested that among patients who attempted suicide parental loss during child-hood is more common than among patients who have not attempted suicide. However among successful suicides a higher rate of early parental death was not found when compared with controls. The precise relationship of early parental death to suicide and attempted suicide has not been fully resolved.

Q4.

Research has shown that shoplifting is more common among women than men and many are either suffering with depression or have an incipient depression and they are more likely to have a history of psychiatric hospitalisation than controls. It has been suggested that there may be an unconscious desire to get apprehended and punished and that this may be an attempt to expiate a feeling of guilt or unworthiness that sometimes accompanies a depressive illness. In contrast to women, male shop lifters are less likely to be depressed but are more likely to be recidivistic. Lack of concentration common among depressives and also found in the mentally well probably results in inadvertent or unintentional shoplifting in supermarkets. Adolescents may shoplift in groups or packs at certain stages of their development.

Q5.
E.C.T. may have a place in the treatment of this patient, because of the endogenous features of his illness, especially if he does not respond to hospitalisation, socialisation and antidepressants and if his suicidal intent persists.

Q6.
All the theories are based on an assumed beneficial therapeutic effect and although the concensus of recent controlled trials suggests a beneficial effect the controversy on the efficacy of E.C.T. continues. Among psychoanalytical theories is the 'regression hypothesis' which suggests that E.C.T. produces a regression of behaviour to the infantile or even the prenatal levels and the Freudian states of psychosexual development are reactivated with beneficial effect. There is also the 'fear hypothesis' which suggests that it is fear of the treatment rather than the treatment itself which is beneficial. The 'punishment hypothesis' suggests that the patient regards the treatment as a form of punishment administered by a strict but forgiving father figure and once the treatment is concluded guilt and fear are resolved. There is also a group of theories based on the suggestion that the treatment-induced amnesia is responsible for the beneficial effects. The amnesia is usually greatest for events coming immediately before treatment and as the symptoms of the illness are recent they are likely to be influenced by the amnesia. It is also suggested that amnesia helps to 'depattern' or break up old undesirable patterns of thinking and behaviour. Other theories have emphasised the shock aspect of the treatment and suggest that the patient gets a psychological jolt which brings him face to face with healthy reality. The 'neural consolidation theory' suggests that E.C.T. breaks up unhealthy consolidated memory traces. In conclusion, psychological theories continue to accrue, but none are adequate, or are likely to be until a process, or processes, of whatever nature can be confidently implicated as being the cause of endogenous depression.

Q7.

This man should be admitted to hospital because he is probably still suicidal and his depression may need more intensive treatment and observation than can be achieved on an outpatient basis. A course of antidepressants of the tricyclic or tetracyclic group could be prescribed for a period to see if he responds and if there is no response after two to three weeks and he remains miserable then a course of E.C.T. could also be tried. Arrangements should be made for him to attend a day hospital or outpatients department after discharge from hospital for regular supervision. The social worker on the psychogeriatric team may be able to help provide a social or recreational outlet for him such as membership of a club or society and regular visitation by the community psychiatric nurse may be indicated.

Q8.

Apart from anorexia nervosa eating disorders are commonly encountered in psychiatric practice. In endogenous depression appetite is commonly impaired and may be associated with considerable weight loss. In catatonic states and in depressive stupor there may be complete refusal of food and drink. Over-eating and obesity may be found in association with anxiety. Although binge eating may be found in 50 per cent of patients with anorexia nervosa it occurs in people who are suffering neither from obesity nor anorexia nervosa. Various names for this disorder have been suggested including 'binge eating syndrome', 'bulimia', 'bulimia nervosa' and 'bulimiarexia'. In Britain the name 'bulimia nervosa' is used and it is described as characterised by a powerful and intractable urge to eat, the induction of vomiting or the abuse of purgatives to avoid the fattening effect of food, and a morbid fear of becoming fat. Frequently fluctuations of weight of 10 pounds or more due to alternating binges and fasts are noted. The patient is aware that the eating pattern is abnormal and a binge is commonly followed by depressed mood.

Course and management

The patient responded to a course of six E.C.T.'s and his depression completely subsided and his belief that the police were watching him lost its intensity. He was discharged home. He continues with tricyclic antidepressants, is supervised regularly by the community psychiatric nurse and visits outpatients regularly. The prognosis for depression in a man of this age is good as it may respond to treatment, however, suicide is common in depressed people of this age.

Further reading

Brown G W, Harris T, Copeland J R 1977 Depression and loss. Brit J Psychiat 130: 1–18

Bunch J, Barraclough B, Nelson B, Sainsbury P 1971 Early parental bereavement and suicide. Soc Psychiat 6: 200–202

Fairburn C 1982 Binge eating and bulimia nervosa. Smith, Kline and French Publications 4

Gibbens T C N 1981 Shoplifting. Brit J Psychiat 138: 346–347

Miller E 1967 Psychological theories of E.C.T. A review, Brit J Psychiat 113: 301–311

Sainsbury P 1968 Suicide and depression. In: Coppen A, Walk A (eds) Recent developments in affective disorders, Headly Bros, Ashford, Kent, p 1–13

CASE 17

A 35-year-old man is referred to psychiatric outpatients by his general practitioner complaining both of loss of sexual interest in the opposite sex and sexual impotence. He was an illegitimate child and his mother married when he was about two years old. He did not get on well with his stepfather, who worked mainly as a labourer and he found great difficulty in relating to him. His relationship with his mother was also poor and as a child he suffered from enuresis and at the age of six he was admitted into care because he was considered to be 'neglected'. Later he spent time in a school for maladjusted children because he had what he describes as an 'uncontrollable temper'. From the age of 13 to 18 he spent periods in five psychiatric hospitals, mainly in adolescent psychiatric departments where he was regarded as a maladjusted youth with an aggressive behaviour disorder. He spent five years in a special hospital after attacking a nurse. After discharge he worked at various jobs and was arrested and charged twice for drunk and disorderly behaviour, but there was no overt aggressive or violent behaviour. Psychosexually he claims to be heterosexual at present. His psychosexual maturing period took place while he was in various institutions in predominantly male company. While in institutions he had two homosexual relationships during which he changed his role from passive to active partner and during this period his masturbatory fantasies were of a homosexual kind. He claims to have had a satisfactory heterosexual relationship including intercourse and had a steady girlfriend for about two years after he left the institution. She was an ex-psychiatric patient and committed suicide about three or four years previously. At present he is unemployed and lives by himself on social security in a council flat. He does odd jobs to supplement his income, smokes about 30 cigarettes a day and drinks very moderately, because he is epileptic. His epilepsy is of the grand mal type and for the last three years he has taken epanutin 400 mg daily and phenobarbitone 120 mg daily. Most of his free time is occupied either in reading, watching television, walking, or repairing electrical equipment for which he appears to have a flair. He has only two or three friends and no girlfriend at present. He describes himself as a friendly, helpful personality, who has outgrown his previous immature antisocial method of behaving and he has no contact with his family as he feels that they have a deleterious effect on him. Apart from his epilepsy there is no relevant medical history. For the last three or four years his interest in the opposite sex and his sexual potency has waned gradually and he cannot relate the onset of his symptoms to any particular incident or event. He had reduced the frequency of masturbation over the same period and says he has not masturbated for many months now and will not get an erection when he does masturbate and he has not attempted intercourse with a female for three or four years. There has not been a morning erection for about two years and he denies that he is homosexual or bisexual at present. On examination he is a pleasant friendly man to talk to. He is not depressed and does not appear unduly concerned about his sexual impotence. He is not aroused by books of a sexually stimulating kind. There are no psychotic features evident and he does not take any unprescribed drugs. On general physical examination he is well and his genitalia appear normal.

Questions

1. What is your formulation on this case?

2. What are the psychiatric and psychological causes of sexual impotence?

3. How important is this patient's epilepsy in the genesis of his sexual symptoms?

4. Would you regard this patient's history of homosexual activity as abnormal?

5. What do you know of the Kinsey Report (1948)?

6. How would you treat this patient?

Answers

Q1.

Loss of sexual interest in the opposite sex and sexual impotence is present in a 35-year-old man separated from his parents since the age of two years and reared in institutions. During his childhood and adolescence he exhibited aggressive and violent behaviour which resulted in his detention in a remand home and subsequently in a special hospital and during his periods in the various institutions he engaged in homosexual activity, but denies that he is homosexual. Since his discharge into the community his general behaviour has improved. He has difficulty in establishing enduring relationships or in holding down jobs which he relates to the fact that employers will not employ him because of his history of epilepsy. His early childhood parental deprivation and the absence of a home atmosphere has probably obstructed mature sexual and personality development. The absence of an early morning erection would suggest an organic basis for his impotence, but a psychological or sexual orientation problem is more likely.

Q2.

Psychiatric causes of impotence include severe depression, anxiety states, chronic alcoholism with secondary malnutrition, dependence on or over medication with barbiturates. It may also be found in association with morbid jealousy and it has also been reported following E.C.T. Psychological impotence (functional impotence) is the most common cause of the condition and is generally regarded as causative when no biological or psychiatric cause is found. From a psychoanalytical viewpoint impotence is due to a castration fear resulting from unresolved childhood incestuous desires for the mother. These desires would be inhibited, so all sexual and coital activity could be prevented by psychological impotence in later life. More recently psychological impotence is viewed as a reaction between sexual endowment and environmental experiences. Whether impotence in adult life is experienced is determined by the interaction of the strength of the sexual desire and the traumatic sexual experiences of early childhood. The characteristics of adult sexual behaviour are thus 'learned upon a genetically determined neuroendocrine framework'. Psychological impotence is divided into early and late onset types. Early onset type is present at the first attempt at coitus and is usually found in individuals with personality disorders or in those of a sensitive or anxious disposition. Frequently there is a history of childhood neurotic traits and poor childhood relationships with parents. Late onset impotence occurs in a previously sexually well adjusted individual and may be a reaction to a current or developing environmental stress and may be acute or insidious in onset. Acute onset may be experienced during the engagement or honeymoon period when the individual is tense or worried or unsure of how his partner will react. It could also follow a trauma such as an operation especially in the perineal or lower abdominal area. Insidious onset impotence may be the end result of an interaction of reduced sexual drive with advancing age and a psychological factor such as the failing sexual attractiveness of the partner, excessive sexual demands by the partner, or of long periods of sexual abstinence due to separation from the partner or involvement in professional duties (barrister's impotence).

Q3.

The patient's history of epilepsy may be a factor worth considering, but is unlikely to be the causative factor. Large doses of anticonvulsants and barbiturates can reduce sexual potency. It is not clear however whether his impotence dates from when he started taking anticonvulsants. Epilepsy (especially temporal lobe epilepsy) has been associated with sexual dysfunction, especially low sexual drive and impotence. This patient, however, does not have temporal lobe epilepsy. A therapeutic trial under observation with a change or reduction in his anti-convulsants and observation of the effect on his potency could be tried, but the results are unlikely to be rewarding.

Q4.

It is difficult to say whether this patient's history of homosexual activity enters the abnormal range. Aspects of the case that suggest it does are that there is doubt about his reliability as a witness, there have been two homosexual affairs and his homosexual activity may be more recent and extensive. Also it must be remembered that this patient is not only impotent but has loss of sexual interest in females, and he appears at interview to be generally unconcerned about his symptoms. Aspects of the case which suggest that his homosexual activity was within the normal range is that some of it took place during his adolescent years which could be regarded as normal developmentally also when he was in an exclusively male environment, without access to female companionship.

Q5.

The Kinsey Report is a study of 4 108 adult American males published in 1948 which reported that over 37 per cent had had adult sexual contact with another man leading to orgasm by the age of 45, also that 4 per cent were exclusively homosexual and 10 per cent were more or less exclusively homosexual for at least three consecutive years and 10 per cent of married men admitted concurrent homosexual experience. The study is a frequently quoted report which while emphasising the incidence and range of homosexual activity has given rise to much discussion on what form of sexual expression in particular settings and age groups can be regarded as within the 'normal' range.

Q6.

It is probably advisable in the first instance to have a few interviews with this patient at outpatients. This would help the patient to feel more at ease and to talk about his problem in more detail. It should become apparent over a period of time firstly whether the patient had intentionally sought referral to a psychiatric clinic or whether it was initiated by the general practitioner without the patient requesting it or being worried about the problem to such an extent that he asked to be referred to a specialist. The degree and nature of his impotence should also become more clear after a series of interviews. The absence of a morning erection would suggest an organic basis, but a psychological cause or a problem with sexual orientation is more likely to be of importance. If the impotence is related to one female only it would suggest that the cause is to be found in the psychosexual relationship with this person, but if the impotence is generalised towards all females as it apparently is in this case then a more general psychosexual explanation should be sought, and treatment should be of a psychosexual nature such as some form of Masters and Johnson therapy. Unless the psychiatrist is experienced in treatment of sexual disorders it may be advisable for him to refer the patient to a colleague experienced in this form of treatment. If it is a problem arising from a disorder of sexual orientation and the patient is worried about it to such a degree that he actively sought referral to a specialist, it suggests that his disorder of sexual orientation is not exclusive and may be amenable to treatment of a psychotherapeutic and/or behavioural kind aimed at reorientation. But if the patient is happy with his particular sexual orientation, then no treatment on these lines is indicated. If it is basically a problem of non-exclusive homosexuality then aversion therapy by pairing chemical or electrical aversive stimuli with photographic, verbal or fantasied stimuli could be tried. Although electrical stimuli are mainly used in Britain because of convenience, chemical stimuli such as paired apomorphine induced nausea appears to be equally effective. It is claimed that up to 40 per cent of patients may be helped either with behavioural or psychotherapeutic methods of treatment. Physical investigation to exclude an organic basis to his problem could be delayed until common more obvious psychological explanations have been excluded.

Course and management

This patient did not keep follow-up appointments regularly. It became apparent that he was not really concerned about the problem.

Further reading

Ansari J M A 1976 Impotence: prognosis (a controlled study). Brit J Psychiat 128: 194–198

Brady J P 1976 Behaviour therapy and sex therapy. Amer J Psychiat 135: 896–899

Hawton K 1982 Major common symptoms in psychiatry, sexual problems. Brit J Hosp Med 27(2): 129–135

Kinsey A C, Pomeroy W B, Martin C E 1948 Sexual behaviour in the human male, Saunders, Philadelphia.

Masters W H, Johnson U E 1970 Human sexual inadequacy, Little Brown, Boston

CASE 18

A 77-year-old woman is referred by her general practitioner to out-patients. According to her daughter, 'she is forgetful and has difficulty in managing at home'. Her father was a labourer and she is the second of five children. She apparently had a happy childhood with no obvious neurotic traits and attended school up to the age of 14, when she got a job doing domestic work. At the age of 19 she married and had three children, two sons and a daughter. There is no psychiatric history for her parents or herself. She describes herself as friendly but the daughter says, 'she has a harsh tongue and can be abusive'. Her husband died 26 years previously, since then she has worked as a part time cleaner. Apparently her confusion was of fairly sudden onset, over a period of a month, about one year previously. Since then it has become progressive and she has become increasingly dependent on her family. She is able to find her way to a local pub where she drinks three to four small bottles of Guinness a day and also walks to a luncheon centre daily. She was seen by a cardiologist a few weeks prior to the interview was found to be fibrillating and is receiving digoxin. She is on no other medication and her health is otherwise good, her blood pressure is 170/90. She is not incontinent and can feed and dress herself. On examination she is confused, disorientated for time and place, knows nothing of current affairs, nor can she name any prominent public figures. She is able to recall the names of members of her family and her address. Her remote memory is better than her recent memory. She cannot retain new information. She is not depressed, but responds to questioning with increased agitation. There is no evidence of functional psychosis.

Questions

1. What are the most likely causes of confusion in a woman of this age?

2. Why do you suggest arteriosclerotic (multi infarct) rather than senile dementia (Alzheimer type)?

3. What is the treatment and management of this patient?

4. Do you know of a possible role for viruses in the etiology of dementia?

5. What general information can be given to anxious relatives of patients with Alzheimer's Disease about the genetic risk to themselves and their children?

Answers

Q1.
The most likely cause of confusion in a woman of this age presenting in this fashion would be either senile (Alzheimer type) or arteriosclerotic (multi infarct) dementia. Other causes of confusion would be depression (pseudo dementia), chronic over-medication with hypnotics and tranquillizers, physical causes such as heart and lung failure, hypothyroidism and nutritional neglect, subdural haematoma. Arteriosclerotic dementia may be the most likely cause here.

Q2.
It is difficult to distinguish between arteriosclerotic and senile dementia especially in advanced cases and there is considerable overlap both in pathology and clinical presentation. Up to 20 per cent of patients have pathology suggestive of both conditions. The findings of fairly quick onset of confusion in this case, the cardiovascular abnormalities, and the general preservation of social functioning would suggest arteriosclerotic dementia. She may have had a subclinical cerebral infarct due to an embolus.

Q3.
This patient should be maintained in the community, with support from the family, social services, also psychiatric and para-medical support as appropriate, such as arrangements to attend outpatients or a psychogeriatric day hospital and/or community psychiatric nurse visitation. Encouragement and support for the caring relatives is vital in this case.

Q4.
There is some evidence of a viral etiology in certain dementias. Creutzfeldt — Jacob Disease — a rapidly progressive dementia occurring in middle age has been transmitted from man to primates and it has been proposed that cytomegalovirus (CMV) infection may be implicated in Alzheimer's Disease. There is also evidence that 'scrapie' a form of 'dementia' in sheep is of viral origin. However a genetic pre-disposition may be essential and Alzheimer's disease may be a classic example of the relationship between genes and viral diseases.

Q5.

Essential to genetic counselling is a detailed family history of the occurrence of the disease in the family. Families with multiple cases have a higher risk than families with an isolated case. The genetic risk is much higher when the index patient's symptoms begin before the age of 65. It has been observed that patients are younger and the disease has a more rapid course in families in which secondary cases occur. Symptoms of dementia occurring after the age of 70 carry little genetic risk for close relatives. When symptoms appear before the age of 65 and another relative has had the disease the risk is considerable. When a proband and a parent are affected nearly half the siblings eventually become demented.

Course and management

It was concluded that this patient was suffering from predominant multi infarct dementia. She now attends a day hospital three days weekly and has a home help. She is not receiving psychotropic medication. The relatives are supported and encouraged to continue their supportive role. The prognosis is of course poor and the objective of the treatment is to keep her in the community for as long as she is receiving adequate care and supervision.

Further reading

Bergman K, Foster E M, Justice A W, Matthews V 1978 Management of the demented elderly patient in the community. Brit J Psychiat 132: 441–449

Corsellis J A N 1977 Supplement. Age and ageing 6: 20–29

Davison A N 1978 Supplement. Age and ageing 7: 139–140

Hachinski V C, Lassen N A, Marshall J 1974 Multi infarct dementia, a cause of mental deterioration in the elderly. Lancet 2: 207–209

Harris R 1982 Genetics of Alzheimer's disease. Brit Med J 284: 1065–1066

CASE 19

A 57-year-old man was diagnosed as suffering with schizophrenia when he was first admitted to a psychiatric hospital in 1952. Since then he has had a total of seven admissions to three hospitals and has been in hospital now continually for 11 years. When he originally presented he felt people were against him, were talking about him and could read his mind. He showed little emotion, was rather affectless and had auditory hallucinations and very little insight. Both his parents were mentally well, his father was a labourer and he is described as having a happy childhood. He was an average scholar at school which he left at 14. He succeeded in joining the army at the outbreak of war even though he was only 16 years old and was wounded in the knee and invalided out. He got a job as a machine operator which he held down for 10 years. There is a pronounced history of psychiatric illness among two of his siblings; one sister committed suicide while depressed and a brother was diagnosed as suffering with schizophrenia. He is married with two children, both described as mentally well. His medical history is not relevant. Premorbidly his personality was described as kind, gentle, co-operative, very willing to please, but not showing much ambition, drive or initiative. Symptoms of schizophrenia began to appear in 1950. Over the years he has had many courses of E.C.T. comprising about 6 E.C.T.'s per course and this has usually been effective in treating him when he becomes depressed and withdrawn, he has also been treated with phenothiazines and his present medication is orphenadrine 100 mg t.d.s., trifluoperazine 5 mg t.d.s, and thioridazine 25 mg t.d.s. On examination he is a large well built balding man, clean in appearance, pleasant and eager to please. He is subservient in attitude quite frequently using the word 'Sir', he is not depressed, there are no obvious florid psychotic features evident, but he is rather bland, lacking in spontaneity and drive. There is no cognitive deficit. The charge nurse describes him as good ward worker, who does not wish to leave the ward to work and is very helpful to other patients running errands for them. He visits the wife who lives close by the hospital. The wife is unwilling to have him home as she suffers with depression.

Questions

1. What is the present problem with this man?

2. Which patients are particularly vulnerable to institutional neurosis?

3. What causes institutional neurosis?

4. Has his numerous courses of E.C.T. and his medication a causative role in his present condition?

5. How may institutional neurosis be prevented?

6. How would you manage this patient?

Answers

Q1.
Although this man is at present symptom free it is likely from his history that he suffers with schizophrenia. His main problem at present however is that he has developed institutional neurosis and does not wish to leave hospital.

Q2.
Institutional neurosis is predominately a problem of chronic schizophrenic patients who spend long periods in hospital, but any patient remaining in an institution for a long period is vulnerable.

Q3.
The total caring environment that exists in many hospitals blunts initiative, spontaneity and drive and is conducive to the development of institutional neurosis. Patients with this condition have marked incapacity and their dependency is great and it is most likely that many of the deficits found result from a disease process, especially chronic schizophrenia, and are unlikely to be cured by rehabilitative measures alone. Despite earlier enthusiasm for quick discharge many schizophrenic patients are still becoming new long stay patients.

Q4.
It has been suggested, but awaits confirmation, that large numbers of E.C.T.'s may result in permanent cognitive deficits and neuroleptics may cause widespread damage to the nervous system, especially if used in the long term. However, there is no evidence of

this here, and it is likely that this man's condition is predominately due to the deficits resulting from schizophrenia.

Q5.

It may not be possible to prevent institutional neurosis fully especially in schizophrenic patients who need frequent hospitalisation. Emphasis should be placed on discharging the patient as soon as possible from hospital. While in hospital emphasis should be placed on ensuring that the patient has contact with the outside world, that periods of enforced idleness are minimised, that the staff are not domineering or bossy, that contact is maintained with relatives and friends and that the occupation or prospects for employment are not lost.

Q6.

This patient is grossly incapacitated and institutionalised, and rehabilitation will have to be gradual. Firstly he should if possible be transferred to another ward. His role as 'ward worker' should cease, and he should be referred to an industrial therapy or occupational therapy unit for occupation outside of the ward setting. Then if he progresses satisfactorily he should be transferred to a hostel, preferably a patient's hostel associated with the hospital and sheltered employment sought for him in the community while he stays in the hostel. The outlook for this man is not very good as he is severely handicapped and the wife does not wish to have him home, or discharged from hospital.

Course and management

The patient refused and/or was unable to co-operate with rehabilitative endeavour. The prognosis for the foreseeable future is poor.

Further reading

Barton R W 1976 Institutional neurosis, 3rd edn, Bristol Wright,

Cunningham Owens D G, Johnstone E C 1980 The disabilities of chronic schizophrenia — their nature and factors contributing to their development. Brit J Psychiat 136: 384–395

Friedberg J 1977 Shock treatment, brain damage and memory loss; a neurological perspective. Amer J Psychiat 134: 1014–1019

Mann ,S, Cree W 1975 The 'new long-stay' in mental hospitals. Brit J Hosp Med 14: 56–63

CASE 20

A lady of 80-years is referred by her general practitioner to psychiatric outpatients, complaining of numerous aches and pains and that her son and daughter-in-law with whom she lives and her doctor do not take her seriously. She is a widow of 22 years duration and has two children. As far as she can recall she had a happy childhood and was reasonably good at school. Her father was a tradesman and her mother died when the patient was aged 16. There is no history of psychiatric illness in the family background. At the age of 15 she got her first job and has worked mainly at clerical work. She married at the age of 22 and described the marriage as a very happy one. For the preceding 11 years she has lived with her son and daughter-in-law, who have no children and both go out to work. There is no previous psychiatric history and she describes herself as normally a very happy person, but is sensitive and inclined to worry a lot. She is interested in crochet, reading, knitting, but complains that 'due to my poor eyesight I cannot now do these things'. She has been physically well up to seven years ago when she fractured her hip and had it pinned. She had a good result up to about a year ago when she said 'it began to give trouble but the surgeon did nothing about it'. She does not smoke and drinks very modestly. She complains of a burning pain in the back of her head, of pains in the back, in her abdomen and in her limbs, of waking up in the middle of the night with pins and needles in the limbs and feeling as if her body is a field of pain, of poor vision so that she finds it difficult to do tasks in the house, and of constipation. She complains of feeling depressed but relates this intimately to her physical state and says 'if only they would talk to me rather than at me, and my doctor is so busy he has no time for me and he will not give me a thorough examination, he keeps telling me I can see when I cannot'. Her appetite is good but she has difficulty in getting off to sleep and wakes early, she has never considered killing herself, but does feel lonely in the house all day. At interview she is a tearful, depressed, agitated woman who relates all her problems to her numerous physical complaints and lack of understanding by her relatives and her general practitioner. She is neat and tidy and looks remarkably well, there are no psychotic features evident and there is no evidence of cognitive impairment. On physical examination the patient appears to be well and can walk about the consulting room quite readily and does not appear to have difficulty with her vision. There was shortening of about one to two inches on the leg which had been operated on.

Questions

1. What is your formulation on this case?

2. What is your concept of hypochondriasis as a distinct clinical entity?

3. How important is this woman's home situation in the genesis of her symptoms?

4. What effect is this woman's symptomatology likely to have on her relatives and her doctor?

5. Apart from hypochondriasis what other ways may affective illness in the elderly present?

6. Is depression in the elderly a forerunner of dementia?

7. How would you treat this patient?

8. What do you understand by the term 'abnormal illness behaviour'?

Answers

Q1.

This is a case of severe depression probably predominately endogenous in type, with secondary hypochondriasis in an 80-year-old woman in good general health, of good intelligence level and personality and without a psychiatric history. Her symptoms have given rise to considerable friction in the home, which in turn has tended to exacerbate her symptoms, and make her conclude that her relatives and her doctor do not 'take her seriously'. The symptoms may be further exacerbated by the fact that she is at home alone all day, unoccupied, ruminating about her health while her relatives are at work.

Q2.

There is considerable discussion on the concept of hypochondriasis as a distinct clinical entity, it is agreed by some that it exists independently, and by others that it is invariably found as a symptom complex of another psychiatric disorder especially depression. It may also be viewed as a neurotic reaction state or a psychotic disorder depending on the intensity of the symptoms. In the Diagnostic and Statistical Manual of the American Psychiatric Association it is defined as a neurotic disorder 'dominated by preoccupation with the body and with fear of presumed diseases of various organs. The fears persist despite reassurance and there are no losses or distortion of function'. These patients are regarded as having a psychotic disorder if the hypochondrical symptoms are of delusional intensity or if there is functional incapacity. The term primary hypochondriasis is used when the condition is encountered unrelated to another psychiatric condition and secondary when it is encountered in the context of another psychiatric state. Although cases of primary hypochondriasis have been described, secondary hypochondriasis in the setting of an affective illness, especially in the elderly is by far the most common type encountered and this is the concept entertained by most psychiatrists.

Q.3
This woman's home situation has probably an important deleterious influence on her symptoms in three ways. Firstly, she is at home all day by herself with nothing to occupy her mind as she claims that she cannot read or go out by herself due to her poor vision so it is likely that she will become morbidly introspective and so exacerbate her symptoms. Secondly, because her son and daughter-in-law do not understand the basis of her complaints and continually admonish her or accuse her of 'putting it on' she will be inclined to react with some acute or dramatic symptoms to gain their respect and attention and of course in the process only alienate herself more from them and from her general practitioner. Thirdly, hypochondriasis can be viewed psychodynamically as a method of shifting anxiety away from interpersonal conflict on to a less threatening concern with bodily function. It is likely that this patient's symptomatology would be productive of considerable ill feeling and conflict within the family setting, and may be a maladaptive method of dealing with familial interpersonal conflict.

Q4.
It is likely that this woman's symptomatology will eventually influence the relatives and the doctor to reject her. The result of this rejection is that the relatives may pay increasingly less attention to her complaints and may make her feel unwelcome in the home. Similarly the general practitioner may become impatient and less

sympathic to her, and should symptoms of an organic basis arise they may not receive the attention they warrant.

Q5.
Depression in the elderly may also present with agitation, restlessness, shop-lifting, paranoia and aggression, guilt feelings, and feelings of unworthiness, nihilistic delusions and symptoms suggestive of cognitive disturbance. There is considerable overlap in symptoms between the reactive and endogenous types of depression and between depression in the adult and in the elderly and it is important to know that some investigations suggest that the above symptom patterns may not be age related.

Q6.
It was a commonly held view of earlier psychiatrists that depression in the elderly may be a forerunner of dementia and this view probably arose from the observation that elderly depressed patients exhibited some cognitive impairment. Research however has not validated this view and has shown that senile (Alzheimer type) or multi infarct dementia did not occur more frequently among elderly depressed patients than in age matched controls.

Q7.
As this patient is not suicidal she could be treated on an outpatient basis. Antidepressant tablets of the tricyclic or tetracyclic type and preferably those described as having minimal cardio-toxic effects could be prescribed. Concurrently she should attend a psychogeriatric day hospital to provide a social and diversional outlet for her and to enable staff to monitor her progress. A thorough physical examination with detailed review of her medical history and of the investigations she has had should be carried out to ensure that there is no organic basis to her symptoms or need to refer for further investigations or opinions. This would also be reassuring to the patient. If the response to antidepressants is unsatisfactory after two to three weeks, then another antidepressant could be tried or she could have a course of E.C.T. With the patient's permission the help of the family in managing the patient should be sought and the nature of her illness explained to them. After the patient has improved she should continue to take antidepressants for a period of from three to six months and then they could be omitted to see how she progresses.

Q8.
The concept of 'abnormal illness behaviour' was formulated in the

late 1960s from sociological studies of the sick role. People may respond to a noxious stimulus in many possible ways varying from a stoical acceptance to hypochondriasis. The desirable response would be one which attracts the attention of the physician and results in removal of the stimulus and restoration of health. In 'abnormal illness behaviour' the object is care rather than cure. Their abnormal illness behaviour is effective in securing care, and this care is so acceptable to the patient that the behaviour which secured it becomes established and difficult to eradicate. Abnormal illness behaviour may result from stress and may present in hypochondrical or hysterical overlay and may be the patient's only way of dealing with problems of daily living. Abnormal illness behaviour is frequently observed in association with established chronic organic disorders, for example the care and attention from doctors and friends which is directed on chronic sufferers such as those with trigeminal neuralgia or other painful conditions, is sorely missed when the cause of suffering is removed by operation or other effective treatment. In this context there have been reports of suicide or attempted suicide after the restoration of sight.

Course and management

The patient showed minimal response to tricyclic antidepressants over a three week period. She then received six E.C.T.'s and improved remarkably, affective and hypochondrical symptoms subsided, and she now attends a psychogeriatric day hospital three days weekly. The prognosis for this type of patient is frequently quite good, many of them responding to antidepressant treatment and environmental manipulation.

Further reading

Bebbington P E 1976 Monosymptomatic hypochondriasis, abnormal illness behaviour and suicide. Brit J Psychiat 128: 475–478

Hill O W 1982 Major common symptoms in psychiatry, psychosomatic symptoms. Brit J Hosp Med 27(2): 122–128

Kenyon F E 1976 Hypochondrical states. Brit J Psychiat 129: 1–14

Pilowsky I 1978 A general classification of abnormal illness behaviours. Brit J Med Psychol 51: 131–137

CASE 21

A 48-year-old man is referred for a psychiatric opinion after treatment in casualty for an overdose of tricyclic antidepressants. His father was a cabinet maker and he had a reasonably good relationship with both parents, both of whom died of natural causes. There is one older brother and there is no family history of psychiatric illness in the family background. He was a full term normal he suffered with nocturnal enuresis up to the age of seven. He started school at the age of five and left at 15, having done moderately well, but without taking examinations. After finishing school he worked with his father before joining the army and serving in the war in Korea. At the termination of hostilities he left the army and trained to be a 'solderer with electrical equipment', but has not worked since 1974, due he says 'to difficulty in finding work because of his psychiatric history'. He smokes 20 cigarettes daily and drinks heavily when he can afford it, but denies having an alcohol related problem. There is no history of illicit drug use. His medical history is irrelevant, but he has had six psychiatric hospitalisations. The first was in 1957 when he was treated for depression and was then well up to 1972 when he was re-admitted. There were admissions in 1974 and 1976 and he was admitted twice in 1978. It appears that all these admissions were for depression which was related to environmental stress particularly marital problems, and he had taken three overdoses during the course of these depressions. He describes himself as being normally cheerful and active with an interest in photography. He is heterosexual and has been married three times. The first was at the age of 21, and there were three children by this marriage, but he says they divorced 'because we got fed up with each other'. The children remained with the mother and were reared by her. He next married a girl he met in a psychiatric hospital but this marriage only lasted about a year as he says 'the girl was very ill and I could not manage her', there were no children. He met his third wife three years previously at a dance, he cannot get on with her, and her two teenage children from a previous marriage are described as 'aggressive and violent towards me'. She ordered him out of the home on the day previous to the overdose and told him she intended divorcing him. He claims that were it not for the behaviour of the children, he would make a success of the marriage, but was so depressed by the wife's threat and having nowhere to go that he decided to kill himself. After taking the overdose he was overcome with remorse and drove to casualty, where he informed them of what he had done. On examination he is a healthy, well behaved, well dressed man. He appears depressed and this is intimately related by him to his marital difficulties. There are no psychotic features present and no evidence of cognitive impairment. Sleep and appetite are not grossly disturbed and he probably is not suicidal at present.

Questions

1. What is your formulation on this patient?

2. How may a patient with an overdose of tricyclic antidepressants present?

3. What are the major causes of marital dysharmony?

4. What is your concept of therapy for marital dysharmony?

5. How would you manage this case?

6. Would you very briefly comment from a socio-psychiatric viewpoint on the following statement. 'It is impossible for an Englishman to open his mouth without making some other Englishman hate or despise him'.

7. What distinguishing features between suicide and parasuicide are you aware of?

Answers

Q1.
This is a case of reactive depression secondary to a crisis in an ongoing state of marital dysharmony. The history of two previous marital failures, and of three previous overdose attempts secondary to marital crises suggests that the patient has difficulties in interpersonal relationships, reacts in a negative fashion to stress and may have a marked deficit in his personality. The impulsive aspect of the suicidal attempt and the fact that the patient immediately regretted his action and sought medical help suggests that there is a strong impulsive behavioural pattern in the patient's personality structure and that the suicidal attempt might be more appropriately described

as a parasuicidal act, performed with the intention of drawing attention to his problem and of gaining admission to hospital.

Q2.
The presentation will depend on the size of the overdose, and the newer tricyclic and tetracyclic drugs are claimed to have much larger safety margins between therapeutic and fatal doses. The patient may present with agitation, hyperreflexia, disturbance of temperature regulation, skin reactions, and dilated pupils. Major signs of overdosage include coma and convulsions. Effects on the cardiovascular system may be the most immediately life threatening and they include serious arrhythmias and conduction defects such as supraventricular tachycardia, atrial flutter or fibrillation, ventricular fibrillation and cardiac arrest in asystole.

Q3.
The causes of marital dysharmony are so numerous and interrelated that even the common causes need to be categorised, and placed under such headings as cultural differences, intellectual and physical differences, differing social habits, personality differences, sexual problems, crisis points in marriage and mental illness

   a. Cultural differences include problems presented for a partner living in an alien culture, or by unaccustomed roles and changed status for the sexes, or by religious practices which cannot be espoused and are considered unacceptable.

   b. Intellectual and physical differences are likely to be a problem when the wife is more intelligent or is more highly educated than the husband and has a better earning capacity, this may lead to a feeling of inferiority humiliation and resentment in the male partner. Likewise when the wife is considerably taller than the husband he may become the butt of jokes or become embarrassed.

   c. Differing social habits - they may come from different social backgrounds. If one partner is home loving while the other is outgoing and gregarious, difficulties in compromising may arise. Alcohol may present a problem in this context. If one partner's social life revolves around the pub or he drinks to excess or has an alcohol related problem then life for a partner with little interest in alcohol could become difficult.

   d. Personality difficulties include incompatabilites of personality in the partner, or adverse personality traits such as psychopathic or paranoid features which find expression in arguments or violence.

e. Sexual problems include problems with sexual identity, unacceptable sexual practices or demands, impotence, premature ejaculation, or sexual activity outside marriage.

f. Crisis points in marriage. Marriages experience stressful phases which need to be understood and overcome. These include, the birth of the first child which can be difficult for the male partner, who has to accept second place in the wife's attention; the 'empty nest syndrome' when the last child goes to school or leaves home for good and which may be stressful especially for the female; retirement may be difficult for the male who has not planned for it, and the demands made by an ageing or demented parent-in-law.

g. Mental illnesses. Any psychiatric illness can embarrass the marital situation, especially such illnesses as schizophrenia, manic depressives psychosis, personality disorder and alcohol and other drug dependencies.

Q4.

Therapy for marital dysharmony is aimed at firstly ascertaining if the marriage is viable, and if it is, secondly to ascertain the cause of the friction and influence or eliminate it. If the couple are incompatible or one member is suffering from severe ongoing psychiatric illness or has lost interest in the partner and transferred his affection and sexual drives to another person then the marriage may not be viable and separation and/or divorce may be advisable. If the marriage is viable then the various causes of marital dysharmony can be explored, preferably in the presence of both partners. The successful marriage should have the following characteristics — it should give the partners the feeling that they have someone to love and are loved in return; it should give them a sense of achievement through help in their careers or from pride in parenthood; both partners should feel that their independence, especially financial independence, has not been removed; it should sustain a feeling of equality between the partners and boost their self-esteem. Enquiry should be made as to which of these desirable characteristics are absent, by the therapist who will see both partners regularly. He may use hypnotherapy or abreactive techniques to explore difficult deep rooted problems in the marriage, and he should keep in mind that his role as a marital psychotherapist should be 'to cure sometimes, relieve often and comfort always', and that time very often has a considerable healing role in these marriages which are passing through time limited crisis points. The psychiatrist should not hesitate in referring the couple to marriage guidance and co-operating with them, as these counsellors may have more expertise in dealing with problems of marital dysharmony which are not the result of personality problems or psychiatric illness.

Q5.

As the patient does not appear suicidal he can be treated on an outpatient basis. Firstly frequent interviews to render supportive psychotherapy, explore the problem at the individual level, and help him overcome the immediate crisis, would be advisable. Next if the patient is agreeable, joint interviews with husband and wife should be pursued to ascertain if the marriage has irretrievably broken down or is still viable. If the marriage is viable the various causes of friction should be identified and means of dealing with them discussed with both partners in an ongoing series of interviews. It should become apparent to the therapist over a period of time, which are the important aspects of dysharmony, which parties can make the major contribution towards solving them and whether the aid of a marriage counselling service or some paramedical facility is also needed.

Q6.

This statement was made by George Bernard Shaw in his preface to Pygmalion, and is a characteristically provocative view aimed at highlighting the social differences in English society, and the sense of grievance which existed at the time in the lower social classes, and the disdainful patronising attitude prominent in the higher classes. The boundaries between the various classes have become less clear cut in the last 70 years due to the availability of better educational, social, occupational and health care facilities. However there are still distinct differences not only in social, cultural and recreational patterns between the lower and higher social grades but also in certain prevalences and methods of presentation of medical and psychiatric conditions. Members of a particular social class will be likely to have similar types of employment, be interested in similar types of sporting activities, read the same newspapers, share the same prejudices, have a similar educational status and speak in characteristic fashion which will tend to make them identifiable to others.

The comment of Shaw could also be regarded as highlighting the profound influence of nurture on nature, in determining the individual's characteristics. The family into which he is born, the education he receives, and the philosophy and views of his peers and colleagues will be likely to be more important in determining his life style and behavioural pattern in health and illness than his genetic endowment.

Q7.

Suicide differs from parasuicide in that the suicide rates are declining in recent years while the parasuicide rates were increasing up to recently but now appear to have peaked and suicide is more common among middle age males in the upper social classes while parasuicide is more common among young females in the lower social classes. Also suicide is more directly related to individuals with psychiatric illness especially psychotic depression or with terminal physical illness. Parasuicide is more directly related to individuals with personality disorders or associated with impulsive behaviour related to acute personal stress. Parasuicidal individuals are also more likely to carry out the act in the presence of others and frequently have a history of similar acts. Although suicide and parasuicide are different in a number of ways there is also a close relationship between the two. 41 per cent of completed suicides have a history of parasuicide.

Course and management

The patient was reconciled to the wife and returned home, joint outpatient appointments for exploration of the problem were not kept. The prognosis for the viability of the marriage may not be good, due to the patient's poor personality and the adverse personal relationship between the patient and his stepchildren. Further marital crises with impulsive parasuicidal behaviour cannot be excluded.

Further reading

Crowe M J 1976 Behavioural treatments in psychiatry. In: Granville Grossman K (ed), Recent advances in psychiatry II, Churchill Livingstone, Edinburgh, London

Forrest A D, Affleck J W, Zealley A K (eds) 1978 Companion to psychiatric studies, 2nd edn, Churchill Livingstone, Edinburgh, London, New York, p 543

Kennedy P, Kreitman N, Ovenstone I M K 1974 The prevalence of suicide and parasuicide (attempted suicide) in Edinburgh. Brit J Psychiat 124: 36–41

Ovenstone I M K 1973 The development of neurosis in the wives of neurotic men. Part II, marital role functions and marital tension. Brit J Psychiat 122: 711–717

CASE 22

A 37-year-old man is admitted to hospital by the police after he suddenly went beserek at home and physically attacked his elderly parents, smashed furniture and fought the police. He is unmarried and lives with his 78-year-old father and 70-year-old mother in a flat. The father, now retired, used to work as a caretaker of a dance hall and the mother is described as nervous. He has one sister and one brother both older than the patient. There is no history of psychiatric illness in the family background. He was a full term normal baby and started school at the age of five; as far as can be ascertained there were no childhood neurotic traits. Generally he was near the bottom of the class scholastically, had few friends and left at the age of 15. His first job was as an assistant in an antique shop which he held for six years and subsequently he worked at labouring jobs such as cleaning premises or warehouse work but hasn't worked for four years. He is described by his sister as always rather shy, aloof and strange, can be hostile, abusive and violent, readily takes offence and finds difficulty in making friends. He is heterosexual but has never been able to establish an enduring relationship with a woman, he smokes moderately and occasionally will drink to excess. Since the age of two he has suffered with epileptiform attacks typical of grand mal seizures, and he says that, 'they came on after I suffered from whooping cough'. He is receiving anticonvulsants primidone 250 mg three times daily and epanutin 100 mg three times daily and he has not had a fit for four years. He has had one previous admission to a psychiatric hospital six years previously after he slashed his wrists subsequent to appearing in court for shoplifting. However, apart from knowing when a seizure is likely, he denies any psychological or perceptual disturbances associated with his epilepsy. On the night of admission he says he suddenly got sick and tired of his parents telling him what to do, and started to shout and strike out at his parents and break the furniture, and his sister called the police. Apparently he had been well up to the outburst, did not feel he was going to have a seizure and he had not been drinking. On examination he is a physically fit looking man who appears to be in the low average intellectual range. There is no cognitive impairment or clouding of consciousness, and there is no clear cut perceptual disturbance. He is, however, quite suspicious and on his guard and expresses the opinion that people do not like him. He appears to be subdued rather than depressed and gives the impression that he could be easily roused to anger and is glad to be in hospital. He does not appear to be suicidal. Physical examination is negative.

Questions

1. What is your formulation on this patient?

2. Briefly discuss the following statement. 'This patient has an epileptic personality disorder.'

3. What do you know of the psychiatric aspects of epilepsy?

4. Do you know of any relationship between epilepsy and schizophreniform psychosis?

5. Are the mentally ill more violent than the general population?

6. Is it possible to accurately predict physical violence in the mentally ill?

7. How would you treat this patient?

8. In which psychiatric conditions may stupor occur?

Answers

Q1.

This patient with a long history of epilepsy is probably functioning within the lower intellectual range of normality, and may be best described as suffering from a personality disorder. This is characterised by gross sensitivity and readiness to take offence, a low frustration level, a history of violence and difficulty in relating to or establishing relationships with others. These aspects of his personality, while probably not predominately due to his epilepsy may have to some degree been exacerbated by it. His violent outburst may have been an overreaction to a frustration.

Q2.

Considerable discussion has existed for many years on whether there is a separate personality type, moulded predominantly by the epileptic process. This postulated epileptic personality has been described as 'touchy, quarrelsome, aggressive, pedantic, egocentric, religiose and circumstantial'. Although a small percentage of epileptics, usually those with a chronic disorder, exhibit this picture, as does the patient in question, it is generally agreed that it is more related to multiple associated handicaps rather than exclusively to the epileptic process. These handicaps include chronic effects of anticonvulsant therapy, difficulty at school, difficulties in getting and holding employment and accommodation and of course the epilepsy may be but a symptom of underlying brain damage which in itself could have an adverse effect on personality. The possibility that the epileptic process itself may have an initiating and/or on-going deleterious effect on personality has not yet been fully excluded.

Q3.

The psychiatric aspects of epilepsy are commonly divided into three groups, mainly disorders of consciousness, disorders of mood and finally psychoses of schizophreniform type. Confusional states are usually precipitated by a fit and are far more common in idiopathic epilepsy than in temporal lobe epilepsy. The patient will appear confused, will perform purposeless acts, may be paranoid, aggressive and truculent and the behaviour may last from a few hours to weeks. Epileptic furor and fugue states do not appear to be as common as believed. Disturbances of mood in the form of anxiety or depression may be observed in the epileptic as a prodrome or briefly as an aura to a seizure. Long lasting depressive episodes are seen and depression may be the commonest formal diagnosis on admission of the patient to a psychiatric hospital. Suicide may be a serious risk with these patients as they have ready access to large quantities of anticonvulsants.

Q4.

The relationship of schizophreniform psychosis to epilepsy is unclear and much discussed. Discussion has mainly been concerned with the question of whether any association is coincidental or causal and of course temporal lobe epilepsy has received most attention. Epileptic fits occur in patients with schizophrenia and among the functional psychoses the greatest percentage of abnormal E.E.G.'s is to be found in schizophrenia, indeed, it has been possible to separate at a statistically significant level the tracings of schizophrenic patients from depressed patients. The more recent studies suggest that there is a causal relationship especially between temporal lobe epilepsy and schizophrenia. It has also been observed that the schizophreniform psychosis is associated mostly with E.E.G. abnormalities in the left temporal lobe. However, it must be remembered that the type of schizophrenia which epileptic psychoses most resemble is paranoid schizophrenia and this is the variety which is probably least clear cut and has the best prognosis. The ability to co-operate with others and respond emotionally to them is better preserved in the epileptic psychoses than in schizophrenia. Difficulties in delineating the boundaries of schizophrenia itself adds to the confusion.

Q5.

It has been generally believed that the mentally ill are not only possessed of super-human strength but are more violent than the general population. However there is little evidence to support the belief that the mentally ill as a group are particularly violent, and in general the underlying personality is of more importance in determining whether a violent act is perpetrated, than the illness from which the patient suffers. Certain types of psychiatric patients may be characterised by violent behaviour, such as patients described as psychopathic or personality disordered, those who abuse or are dependent on alcohol or other drugs, patients with morbid jealousy, and some schizophrenic patients especially those with marked paranoid symptomatology.

Q6.

At present it is not possible to accurately predict when or where a particular patient will exhibit violence and few psychiatrists believe they can do so. A violent act is frequently the end result of a complex interaction between the personality of the patient, the illness from which he suffers and the frustrations existing in the environment in which he lives. An age under 50 combined with a history of frequent violence are the only guidelines of any use in predicting violent behaviour and these are also generally inaccurate. Nevertheless violent behaviour by psychiatric patients is overpredicted because the error to avoid is the one that would incur censure, such as when a patient predicted to be non-violent exhibits violence in public. Thus many non-violent patients are detained in hospital or prison so that the few will not exhibit violence.

Q7.

It is probably advisable to admit this patient to hospital for further assessment because return home may re-expose him to some frustration there which would trigger off further violence towards the elderly parents. There would be an opportunity to re-assess his epilepsy and review his medication and it may be possible to prescribe one rather than two anticonvulsants. He should be referred for psychological and occupational assessment and the possibility of him being discharged to a group home or hostel and of working in a sheltered environment should be explored. Alternatively he may eventually be discharged home to attend a day hospital or an industrial therapy unit daily depending on how he responds to treatment. If the patient exhibited ongoing serious violence in hospital then treatment in a special ward, the use of tranquillisers and possibly the advice of a forensic psychiatrist may be indicated who could advise on general management and on whether admission to a special semi secure unit for the treatment of violent patients is indicated.

Q8.

Stupor has been described as a state of complete psychomotor inhibition with retention of consciousness. In psychiatric practice stupor may be seen in severe affective disorders, schizophrenic catatonic states and other less common conditions collectively described as 'psychogenic stupor'. Severe psychiatric stupor is uncommon. The type described as depressive stupor usually is seen in the middle-aged and follows a period of increasing psychomotor retardation, although it may come on suddenly after a bereavement. E.C.T. is usually very effective in its treatment. Although catatonic stupor is usually found in association with schizophrenia it cannot be considered synonymous with it. Before the introduction of neuroleptics it was fairly common to see schinzophrenic patients in psychiatric hospitals standing relatively motionless for long periods or exhibiting what was described as 'flexibilitas cerea' or 'automatic obedience' Psychogenic stupor is acute in onset occurs in certain vulnerable individuals in response to traumatic events such as stress under prolonged battle conditions, sexual assault or witnessing a major accident.

Course and management

The patient remained in hospital for approximately one month, there were no further violent episodes and he was discharged to a patient's hostel and works in a sheltered environment and is followed up at psychiatric outpatients.

Further reading

Fottrell E 1981 Violent behaviour by psychiatric patients. Brit J Hosp Med 25: 28–38

Gunn J 1979 Forensic psychiatry. In: Granville Grossman K (ed) Recent advances in clinical psychiatry 3, Churchill Livingstone, Edinburgh, London, p 271–282

Johnson J 1982 Stupor — its diagnosis and management. Brit J Hosp Med
27(5): 530–532

McClelland R 1979 In: Hill, Murray, Thorley (eds), Essentials of postgraduate
psychiatry, Academic Press, London, New York

CASE 23

A 58-year-old woman is admitted to hospital under emergency section of the Mental Health Act (1959) by the police having been found in the street, shouting, crying and banging her head against a wall. The father died at the age of 80, he was a successful business man, and the mother died of an accident at the age of 78; she had a good relationship with both parents. During the last 20 years of her life the mother suffered with bouts of depressive illness. There is one sister two years older than the patient who is well mentally. She describes her childhood as generally unhappy due to various frequent childhood illnesses which interfered with her schooling and at the age of five she was placed in convalescence for one year away from home due to an unspecified illness. Due to her frequent abscences she was below average at school, left at the age of 15 and did a secretarial course and became a secretary. She had the menarche at 13, and had many boy friends before she met her future husband. She got pregnant by him and had an abortion, and married him when she was 26. She describes him as a kind, loving and caring business man, who died of cancer at the age of 56. There is one son aged 29 who is well. She describes herself as a delicate spoiled person who always had, 'my own way as a child by crying', is dependent on others; originally on her father, then her husband, now on her son, she cannot cope with difficulties, 'I go to pieces when events become threatening'. There is no history of drug abuse and she does not drink or smoke. There is no history of relevant physical illness. Up to recently she lived with her son. She says, 'I had my first breakdown needing admission to hospital 11 years ago when I learned of my husband's illness'. Since then she has had 16 admissions to hospital and four private consultations. She relates her present illness to when she was discharged from psychiatric hospital two weeks previously to a new flat which she did not like and was upset because the son declared his intention of marrying a girl of whom she did not approve. Over the ensuing week she became very depressed by these events and began to behave in a noisy attention seeking manner initially in the neighbourhood and subsequently on the high street until she was brought to hospital by the police. At admission she is unco-operative, keeps her eyes firmly shut resists attempts to open them, is moving her arms up and down, sits on a bed when requested to do so then immediately flops backwards. She understands questions and answers briefly but appropriately but sometimes she repeats, 'I can't remember'. There are no psychotic features evident nor evidence of cognitive impairment and she is fully conscious; there is no evidence of abuse of alcohol or drugs or evidence of physical injury, and routine physical investigations are normal. Shortly after admission she became quite mute, refused to co-operate with staff or answer questions although she appeared to be in contact with her environment.

Questions

1. What is your formulation on this patient?

2. Which personality inventories may be of use in elucidating this patient's personality structure?

3. What is your concept of the term 'hysterical personality'?

4. How important as an impediment to personality maturation was this patient's separation from her parents for a year at the age of five?

5. Do you think this patient could be described as a 'borderline personality'?

6. What is the relationship of pre morbid personality to depression?

7. How would you treat this patient?

8. Very briefly what do you understand by 'crisis intervention'?

Answers

Q1.

It is probable that this patient is suffering from reactive depression with histrionic attention seeking behaviour in the setting of a poor pre morbid personality structure characterised by over dependence on others. She tends to make excessive demands on others, originally on her father, then on her husband, and now on her son; and she relates the onset of her psychiatric illness to the loss of her husband on whom she was very dependent. Her present symptoms have been triggered off by moving into a flat she does not like and by the son's expressed intention of marrying, and her behaviour may be directed to some degree at preventing his marriage. Her maladaptive behaviour may have been reinforced by frequent admissions to hospital, where her dependency and attention seeking needs are met.

Q2.

The hysterical personality is generally described as demonstrative, attention seeking, with rapid short lived mood changes. Hysterical personalities may dress, speak or behave in such a manner that they become the focus of attention, they are self-centred and seem to revel in emotional storms. They have been described as 'craving to appear both to themselves and to others as more than they are and desiring to experience more than they are ever capable of experiencing. The place of genuine experience and natural expression is usurped by a continual stage act, a forced kind of experience'. It is important to note that the majority of hysterical neurotic patients do not have pre morbid hysterical personalities and that there is also discussion on the validity of the concept of hysterical personality as an aggregate of the above traits.

Q3.

There are three major personality inventories which singly or in conjunction could be used to shed further light on this patient's personality. There is the Minnesota Multiphasic Personality Inventory (M.M.P.I.) which is widely used in the United States. There are over 500 responses which can be categorised into scales for example for hysteria and depression. It has been criticised because it is time consuming, it does not allow sufficiently for 'normal' personality variation and has been developed from research on psychiatric populations. The Eysenck Personality Inventory (E.P.I.) is a two dimensional scale measuring extroversion — introversion and neuroticism. A much criticised third scale for measuring psychoticism has been included in an updated version of the Eysenck Personality Inventory. The Middlesex Hospital Questionnaire covers six scales, mainly phobias, obsessions, free floating anxiety, hysteria and somatic anxiety and depression, and gives a profile of six scores. It is easy to use, quickly administered and is popular.

Q4.

It is difficult to say with any degree of accuracy how important parental deprivation is as a factor in producing personality immaturity in the individual case. Personality impairment may arise from poor genetic endowment, adverse biological factors either intra or extrauterine, and poor environmental, educational and social influences. In general faulty or disrupted parental relationships in the early childhood years result in personality traits which make the individual less well adapted to cope with life's problems and may predispose him to neurotic illness or maladaptive responses to stress and anxiety. Proximity to the parents especially the mother is most crucial during the first two to three years of life and it is during these years that the basis of the child's earliest social interactions are laid. Although the patient was not separated until the fifth year of life, nevertheless it could instil anxiety, resentment and insecurity in the developing personality by breaking established bonds and relationships and the patient still regards the separation as traumatic.

Q5.
A controversial population of individuals described as 'borderline states, borderline patients, or borderline personalities' is found mainly in the American Psychiatric literature. They are described as persons with intense affect usually depressive or aggressive, who exhibit bizarre punitive responses on unstructured psychological tests such as the Rorschach but not on structured tests such as the W.A.I.S. They may exhibit marked degrees of dependency and there is a suggestion that borderline persons may have a high incidence of early maternal loss. This patient has some of the criteria for the borderline state, such as depression and intense dependency on others and of course there is the history of early maternal deprivation for a year as distinct from maternal loss.

Q6.
The relationship of pre morbid personality to affective illness is complex, unclear and raises the question of the classification of affective disorder. The view that there are abnormalities in the personalities of patients with affective disorder is widely held. Overall research suggests that the personalities prone to affective illness, may be less likely to cope positively with stress, tend to worry more, have less initiative and drive, may be more sensitive and insecure and are more dependent than normal personalities. These characteristics are probably more valid for the personality likely to present with the neurotic or reactive type of depression than for the personality which presents with depression with endogenous features. Studies using personality inventories on depressive personalities have shown that they score on neuroticism, obsessional state and trait scales. These described personality characteristics are consistent with the major psychological theories of depression such as the psychoanalytical view that depression prone personalities are greatly

dependent on narcissitic overtures derived directly or indirectly from others for maintenance of their self esteem and may employ various techniques, submissive, demanding, or piteous to maintain these overtures. Another theory maintains that the personality prone to depression has an enduring cognitive set of negative attitudes regarding himself and his environment so that he always expects defeat and frustration and tends to regard himself as unworthy. It is likely that the personality profiles of the various depressive sub types differ and research aimed at elucidating these differences will be important in our understanding of depressive illness.

Q7.
This patient will be difficult to treat, because of her poor personality structure, the duration of her psychiatric history, the presence of what she regards consciously or subconsciously as causative or precipitating events, i.e. the son's intent to marry and dissatisfaction with her new accommodation. Her history of many psychiatric hospitalisations which may have led to some degree of institutionalisation as well as reinforcing her maladaptive behaviour patterns in the face of stress would tend to darken the prognosis. She should be discharged from hospital as soon as the immediate crisis subsides and readmission should be resisted. The help of the son in adopting a firm but understanding attitude to the patient should be sought. Attendance at a psychiatric day hospital may fulfil her dependency needs and the help of a crisis intervention team to help her over difficult periods while remaining out of hospital may be useful. Psychotropic medication has probably a minor role to play in her management. The prognosis is poor.

Q8.
Crisis intervention could be best described as a technique used in the practice of preventive psychiatry. The majority of individuals experience crises of various kinds throughout life and cope with them. Certain vulnerable personalities may need assistance in coping and crisis intervention is concerned with the form this assistance should take so that personal confidence results rather than maladjustment and psychiatric dependency. Frequently it is a soft option for psychiatrists to admit to hospital people they contact in crises. It may be far better in the long term for the individual that the crisis should be managed in the setting in which it arose, which is frequently the home, whether it is a suicidal intention, an adverse reaction to bereavement or retirement, or a case of baby or wife battering. Medical and para-medical personnel may need to visit the setting

of the crisis frequently until the acute stage has subsided and a crisis intervention team will facilitate this and also reduce the number of unnecessary admissions to hospital.

Course and management

The patient was discharged after one week, she attends a day hospital and it is planned to deal with her 'crises' in the community rather than in hospital.

Further reading

Caplon G 1964 Principles of preventive psychiatry, Tavistock Publications Ltd, London

Gunderson J G, Singer M P 1975 Defining borderline patients: an overview. Amer J Psychiat 132: 1–10

Hirschfeld R, Klerman G 1979 Personality attributes and affective disorders. Amer J Psychiat 136: 67–70

Mann A, Murray R 1979 Measurement in psychiatry. In : Hill, Murray, Thorley (eds) Essentials of postgraduate psychiatry, Academic Press, London, New York

Rutter M 1972 Maternal deprivation re-assessed, Penguin, London

Walton H J, Presley A S 1973 Use of a category system in the diagnosis of abnormal personality. Brit J Psychiat 122: 259–267

CASE 24

A 26-year-old girl is referred to a psychiatric hospital for admission, after a suicidal attempt by overdosing with Nitrazepam. Her father died when she was aged 13, by committing suicide while depressed; she says he was diagnosed as schizophrenic. Her mother remarried when the patient was 14, and she and her 20-year-old brother live with the parents. There are frequent arguments in the house, mainly due to the stepfather's excessive drinking. The patient was born after a full term normal pregnancy, but as a two year old she had bouts of screaming and was a poor sleeper and experienced many nightmares; otherwise she appeared to have a normal childhood. She attended school up to the age of 16, was an average student and got work as a clerical officer after leaving and continued at this type of work for about six years, but hasn't worked for the last three or four years. She describes herself as introverted, shy, withdrawn and finds difficulty in relating to others. Psychosexually she never experienced the menarche, has persistent amenorrhoea and never had a relationship with a man. She has had five previous psychiatric hospitalisations, the first 13 years ago, the second three years previously, one the previous year and two in the current year. For the previous month the patient believed that the devil was after her. She lay awake at night worried about this and thought that he was tapping on her window. She also heard the voice of a man talking about her and commenting on her actions. At times she felt that she was under the control of the devil, that he was talking through her and had power to inflict pain on her. She thought the best way to escape was to take an overdose and kill herself, but her mother suspected that she had done so, called the ambulance and she was referred to a psychiatric hospital via a casualty department. At interview she is a girl of short stature with poorly developed secondary sexual characteristics and has webbing of the neck. She still hears voices commenting on her behaviour. She has ideas of influence and passivity feelings and thinks someone has the power to control her voice and inflict suffering on her. She is upset by these beliefs, but is not otherwise depressed and is not suicidal at interview.

Questions

1. What is your formulation on this patient?

2. What psychiatric implications of sex chromosome abnormalities are you aware of?

3. What is the dopamine hypothesis of schizophrenia?

4. What is the prognosis for this girl?

5. Briefly how does the British diagnostic concept of schizophrenia differ from that of the United States?

6. What is the drift hypothesis?

7. How would you treat this patient?

8. What is the current view on the role of propranolol in psychiatric treatment?

Answers

Q1.

This is a case of a suicidal attempt in a 26-year-old girl with a long psychiatric history, suffering from florid schizophrenia with Schneiderian first rank symptoms of auditory hallucinations, consisting of the voice of a man talking about her and commenting on her, passivity feelings and delusions of being under the control of the devil. The physical characteristics of the patient such as webbing of the neck, poorly developed secondary sexual characteristics and low stature in association with her psychosexual history strongly suggests that she also has Turner's Syndrome.

Q2.

Chromosomal aberrations are found in 1 per cent of all newborn babies and knowledge of the psychiatric effects of these abnormalities is derived mainly from comparing their prevalence in abnormal series with the prevalence in the general population. Positive sex chromatin is more common among the mentally retarded than in the general population. Experience also shows that the greater the number of excess chromosomes the greater is the mental retardation, so that males with two additional X chromosomes are more retarded than males with only one extra. However, the double X male constitution may be compatible with overall normal intelligence. Sex chromatin positive Klinefelter males are described as being a special kind of personality described as passive-aggressive and tend to be aggressive. It has also been observed that sex chromatin positive males are three times more common in mental hospital populations than in the general population. There is evidence to suggest that males with an extra X chromosome have a greater risk of becoming antisocial than do other males. The lack of an X chromosome in women seems to have far less effect on their mental health than does the presence of an extra X chromosome. The previously postulated relationship of an extra Y chromosome in men with criminality and psychopathy is not now thought to be valid.

Q3.

The dopamine hypothesis proposes that schizophrenia is due to an increased synthesis and/or release of dopamine in the schizophrenic brain. This hypothesis arose from the observation that amphetamine abuse can result in a schizophrenic-like psychosis with ideas of reference and auditory and visual hallucinations. Amphetamine potentiates the action of dopamine both by releasing it into the synaptic gap and preventing its uptake by the neurone. The observation that dopamine was low in the caudate nucleus in Parkinson's disease and that drugs used in the treatment of schizophrenia frequently caused a Parkinsonian like syndrome often in direct ratio to their efficacious effect further supported the dopamine hypothesis. It is postulated that the antipsychotic drugs exert their beneficial effect by blocking post synaptic dopamine receptors and thereby produce a functional dopamine deficiency. It is also interesting to note that increased dopamine concentrations have been found in schizophrenic brains at post-mortem. There is need, however, for further research to validate the hypothesis and this research is ongoing and exciting.

Q4.

The prognosis for this girl is not good. Schizophrenia of poor prognosis is associated with early onset in the middle teens, a history of schizophrenia in first degree relatives, poor sexual and social premorbid adjustment, the lower social classes and the absence of a history of affective illness in the family history or the absence of a marked affective component in the patient's illness. This patient's presentation would satisfy most of these adverse criteria. The course the patient's illness has followed in the previous 10 years, with a total of five admissions to psychiatric hospitals and with four admissions occurring within a three year period augurs unfavourably for the future.

Q5.

The concept of schizophrenia is much broader in the United States than in Britain due mainly to the predominately psychoanalytical approach and to the influence of Bleuler and Meyer. The British concept of schizophrenia is more narrowly based on the approach of Kraepelin and Schneider with the result that in a comparable population of patients the diagnosis of schizophrenia is made twice as frequently in the United States as it is in Britain and would include in the catergory patients likely to be diagnosed as manic depressive or neurotic in Britain or Western Europe. Many American psychiatrists would claim that schizophrenia is a time related diagnosis and that a proportion of patients diagnosed as manic depressive eventually develop overt schizophrenia.

Q6.

The drift hypothesis proposes that schizophrenic patients drift down the social scale, live in the poorer areas of cities or in slums and are found more commonly in the lower social classes because the illness blunts their initiative, drive and economic effectiveness. Support for this view is provided by the observation that the relatives of schizophrenics are in higher status occupations than the patients. The alternate view (social causation hypothesis) proposes that adverse social conditions either cause or trigger off a schizophrenic illness. The drift hypothesis has wider support.

Q7.

Due to the florid aspects of her symptoms and to her distress, it would probably be advisable to admit this patient. Her psychotropic medication should be reviewed, to ascertain if she has medication regularly or if her relapse is associated with inadequate dosage, or unintentional or intentional omission of treatment. While in hospital it is possible to do a therapeutic trial of a range of psychotropic drugs until the preparation and the dosage most effective for her has been ascertained. It is likely that a long acting intra muscular drug with sedative rather than stimulating effects is appropriate. The psychiatric social worker should investigate the home situation, obtain a full history from relatives, which may throw light on aspects of the illness which are not considered important by the patient, but which may be crucial in long term management. As soon as the acute aspects of the illness subside she should attend occupational or industrial therapy and after discharge she should be followed up at outpatients and by the community psychiatric nurse. Attendance at a psychiatric day hospital or work in a sheltered environment may be appropriate. Medication should continue for the long term.

Q8.
Propranolol is accepted as useful in the treatment of anxiety states with prominent subjective somatic symptomatology such as palpitations, tachycardia, and sweating. The initial enthusiasm for propranolol in the treatment of schizophrenia has not been justified. There is no convincing evidence that propranolol is effective in the treatment of schizophrenia, or superior to placebo. When used in conjunction with chlorpromazine the plasma levels of chlorpromazine are significantly increased and this may produce an enhanced therapeutic effect for a specific dose of chlorpromazine.

Course and management

The patient was admitted to hospital and responded to fluphenazine decanoate in moderate dosage and was discharged after five weeks to attend a psychiatric day hospital.

Further reading

Bird E D, Spokes E G, Barnes J, MacKay A U P, Iverson L, Shepherd M 1977 Increased dopamine and reduced glutamic acid decarboxylase and choline acetyl transference acitivity in schizophrenia. Lancet 2: 1157–1158

British Medical Journal 1977 Editorial — First attacks of schizophrenia. Brit Med J 1: 733–734

Forssman H 1970 The mental implications of sex chromosome aberrations. Brit J Psychiat 117: 353–363

Goldberg E M, Morrison S L 1963 Schizophrenia and social class. Brit J Psychiat 109: 785

Leff J 1977 Review article: international variations in the diagnosis of psychiatric illness. Brit J Psychiat 131: 329–338

Peet M, Middlemiss D N, Yates R A 1981 Propranolol in schizophrenia. Brit J Psychiat 139: 112–117

CASE 25

A 37-year-old man is brought to a psychiatric hospital by the police after being arrested while trying to kill himself by touching electric wires in a railway station. He was born in England and his father worked as a railway porter and he was the second of six children. One of the siblings was treated in a psychiatric hospital for alcoholism but there is no further history of psychiatric illness in the family. There was a poor childhood relationship with the parents, his father abused alcohol, and he was admitted into care at the age of five after his mother assaulted him with a sweeping brush and he received extensive bruising. As far as can be ascertained there were no childhood neurotic traits exhibited. He was an average student at school and at the age of 16 he joined a teenage group and was sent to Borstal for shoplifting and petty theft. While in Borstal he claims to have been subjected to homosexual rape on two occasions. Psychosexually he is heterosexual and first had intercourse at the age of 18. He never married but had two relationships with women and fathered a child by each, these children remaining with their mothers. He got his first job at the age of 17 as an apprentice joiner, but he did not keep it very long and since then has had numerous jobs, mainly of a labouring type. Overall he estimates he has spent about six years in jail for shoplifting, petty theft and failing to pay maintenance for his children. His past medical history is irrelevant and he says he got 'caught in a rut and missed out on life'. He smokes 20–30 cigarettes daily and says he would 'drink a bottle of whisky a day if I could afford it', but denies that he is dependent on alcohol and when he cannot afford it he claims it does not worry him. However, he claims to 'need diazepam' 10 mg three times daily to control my nerves'. He has taken this dosage for a couple of years, and denies taking any other drugs. If he omits diazepam he claims 'I feel I'm going insane, everything becomes unreal and my mind speeds up and I cannot sleep'. He had five previous psychiatric admissions to different hospitals over the previous five years, these have been for treatment of depression with suicidal attempts such as three overdoses with drugs and one attempt by slashing his wrists. While in prison he has also received psychiatric treatment which he describes as psychoanalysis, which consisted of 'talking to a psychiatrist for about one hour per week'. This lasted for about four months and he says he did not benefit from the treatment. At interview the patient is intoxicated and smells of alcohol, he is aggressive and truculent and no history is available at admission. The following morning he is calm, there are no obvious withdrawal effects from alcohol, he appears to have insight into his condition, there are no psychotic features evident and he volunteers the above history. He is not depressed and states that his suicidal attempt occurred mainly because he was under the influence of alcohol at the time. General physical examination and investigations are negative.

Questions

1. What is your formulation on this case?

2. What are your views on benzodiazepine dependence?

3. Which criteria would guide you in selecting patients likely to benefit from long term psychoanalysis?

4. Would you very briefly, comment critically on the following statement 'Psychoanalysis has made a greater contribution to the advance of literature and the arts than to psychiatry'?

5. Do you know of any personal, social or clinical characteristics of parents who batter their children?

6. How would you treat this patient?

Answers

Q1.
This young man has a long history of psychiatric hospitalisation and imprisonment and is in all probability suffering from a pronounced personality disorder with marked psychopathic traits. His poor early childhood relationship with his parents and his long history of institutionalisation are major contributing factors to his poor personality formation. It is likely that he is at least psychologically dependent on diazepam and may have a greater alcohol related problem than he admits to. The suicidal attempt appears to have been impulsive and was probably facilitated by the fact that he was intoxicated at the time. It is not clear how far his attempt could be described as 'a cry for help'. Aspects of this patients's case which suggest that the prognosis is poor is that he is socially isolated, is homeless and without employment and although entering his late

30s has so far shown little evidence to suggest that he can adequately cope with life and its difficulties.

Q2.

Benzodiazepines are probably the most widely used drugs in the history of psychopharmacology and generally accepted as most useful substances in the treatment of anxiety and phobic states and psychosomatic conditions and as an adjunct to other psychotropic drugs. Recent reports have suggested that their potency especially diazepam in inducing psychological and physical dependence especially in long term users is far greater than was believed for many years. It has been established for many years that sudden withdrawal of patients from high dosages of benzodiazepines produces distinct physical and psychological withdrawal symptoms. Recent reports suggest that withdrawal from more modest therapeutic doses which have been used over long periods produces a withdrawal syndrome characterised by psychological and physical features such as anxiety, agitation, insomnia, restlessness, muscle twitching, dizziness and palpitations. These symptoms are relieved by retaking benzodiazepines and are only of a few days duration if the patient continues to abstain from the drug. However in each inidvidual case one must take the overview and in considering their continued use balance the problem of dependence against the disabling effects of chronic anxiety on the patient and the likelihood that should the benzodiazepines be withheld the patient may substitute a more dangerous drug or have recourse to alcohol. Recent reports suggest that prolonged diazepam use may result in brain damage.

Q3.

Selecting patients likely to benefit from long term psychoanalysis (which may last from three to six years) requires considerable discretion. Many factors will have to be considered including, of course the psychiatric illness and in general, neuroses, personality disorders and sexual problems benefit rather than psychoses. The age of the patient is important and generally those under 40 do better than those in the older age groups. The patient should be willing to form a long term contractural arrangement with the therapist and be a person likely to keep appointments, and co-operate with treatment arrangements. At least a normal intellectual level is desirable and the patient should be capable of coping emotionally and intellectually, with insights into his personal and interpersonal life, resulting from the analysis, which might be difficult to accept, and should be a person capable of psychosocial adaptation.

Q4.

This view has arisen mainly because of the difficulty experienced in establishing psychoanalysis as a scientific method of psychological exploration and as an effective therapeutic instrument. For the first 50 years of its existence it has depended for respectability on description and anecdote while a large part of the psychiatric world, resisting the eclectic approach, favoured organic or behavioural methods of treatment. Psychoanalysis has always been a popular topic for the cartoonist and the informed public, and writers and artists have so attempted (successfully some would say) to enrich their creations with deep psychological meaning based on the tenets of psychoanalysis, that a new form of literary and fine art resulted. More recently psychoanalysts are using research data to scrutinize their concepts and treatment results and are attempting to define and monitor the relationships between in-depth analysis and focal psychotherapy and explore the relationship between personality maturation behaviour therapy and psychoanalysis. This research in psychotherapy is likely to result in psychoanalysis being more widely respected while having a more defined format.

Q5.

It has been shown in investigations of the parents of battered babies that pre-marital pregnancy and illegitimacy, absence of the child's father, marital dysharmony and rejecting attitudes towards the child are precursors of baby battering. The housing situation of the parents is poor, and they are more likely to be in the lower social groups, however, their weekly expenditure on food compares well with families in the same social groups. Social isolation and lack of kinship support is also characteristic of battering parents. There is a high frequency of psychopathy in the fathers and neuroticism and subnormality in the mothers and the parents may themselves have been victims of parental violence as children.

Q6.

The patient should be admitted for further assessment (as he may still be suicidal) and to assess his degree of dependence on drugs and alcohol. If he is willing, diazepam may be reduced and withdrawn but it is probably better not to make an issue of his abandoning diazepam use. If he is depressed then this should be treated with drugs and/or electro-convulsive treatment as appropriate. If the patient improves and wishes further help then the possibility of referral to an assessment unit to ascertain the type of occupation most appropriate could be considered. Social intervention to provide an after-care hostel and sheltered employment may be indicated as well as follow up at psychiatric outpatients.

Course and management

The patient improved after two days hospitalisation, he was not depressed, no psychotropic medication was prescribed. The diazepam was reduced to 5 mg three times daily, but he did not wish to omit it completely. He had an alcohol related problem in the form of episodic excessive drinking bouts and expressed the intention of abstaining from alcohol in the future. Plans were formulated for his discharge to a hostel specialising in patients with alcohol problems and for him to attend psychiatric outpatients. Consensus opinion favoured the view that he suffered essentially from poor personality development due mainly to an inadequate family background and long periods of imprisonment and institutionalisation.

Further reading

Kelk N 1977 Is psychoanalysis a science? A reply to Slater. Brit J Psychiat 130: 105–111

London P, Klerman G L 1982 Evaluating Psychotherapy. Amer J Psychiat 139(6): 709–717

Slater E 1975 The psychiatrist in search of a science: III The depth psychologies. Brit J Psychiat 126: 205–224

Smith S M, Hanson R, Noble S 1974 Social aspects of the battered baby syndrome. Brit J Psychiat 125: 568–582

Tyrer P 1980 Dependence on benzodiazepines. Brit J Psychiat 137: 576–577

CASE 26

A 78-year-old lady is admitted to hospital for treatment of depression which has not responded to outpatient treatment with tricyclic antidepressants, perhaps because she has been unreliable in taking her medication regularly. She was born in London, the father was a labourer and there were two other siblings, a boy and a girl, both older than the patient. Overall she had a happy childhood, there is no history of psychiatric illness in the family background. She attended school up to the age of 14, was a moderately good scholar and after leaving school she got a job in a factory and remained there for six years until she met her husband, who worked as a lorry driver. Her marriage has been a happy one, there are three daughters, all married with families of their own. The husband is still alive and the children keep in contact with the parents who live in a small three bedroom house. She is normally a shy sensitive person, has a small circle of friends and her social outlet and recreation takes place mostly in the home setting, where she watches television, knits and reads women's magazines. She does not drink or smoke and there is no previous history of psychiatric illness. For the past 10 years the patient has suffered from Parkinson's disease and is taking L-dopamine tablets one three times daily. According to the relatives she has been unwell since the death six months previously of a sister she was close to, which left a great vacuum in her life and she has never really got over it. Over the previous three or four months she has become withdrawn, her appetite has deteriorated and she has lost over a stone in weight, her sleep is disturbed and she is inclined to awaken quite frequently during the night. She has also become more dependent on the husband and she resents this as she was always a very independent woman. At interview she is a poor historian and the history is obtained from relatives. The patient has marked psychomotor retardation, she remains relatively immobile and answers questions in a monosyllabic fashion. There is no cognitive disturbance and there are no psychotic features evident and she does not admit to feeling suicidal. Physical examination shows Parkinson's disease and routine physical investigation shows that she has a haemoglobin level of 8.5 grams per 100 mls., with a microcytic hypochromic cell pattern.

Questions

1. What is your formulation on this patient?

2. How important was this woman's bereavement in the etiology of her illness?

3. Do you know of any association between Parkinson's disease and psychiatric illness?

4. Has this woman's low haemoglobin level contributed to her symptomatology?

5. How reliable are elderly psychiatric patients in taking their medication?

6. What do you know of the 'monoamine hypothesis' of affective illness?

7. What are the short-comings of this hypothesis?

8. How would you treat this patient?

Answers

Q1.
This patient with Parkinson's disease is probably suffering from an endogenous type of depression with disturbance in appetite, sleep and motivation, in the setting of a good previous personality who has coped admirably with day to day problems upto the onset of her depression. The death of her sister may have been an important precipitating factor in her illness and it is quite possible that the initial grief reaction to this loss may have with time assumed the characteristics of an endogenous depression. The prognosis with uninterrupted antidepressant therapy is probably good.

Q2.
It is difficult to say how important this woman's bereavement was in the causation of her illness. It is established that important life events antedate depressive illness and death of a close relative is a most important life event. Normally a grief reaction which resolves with time is to be expected after the loss of a close relative, and three phases are described for this reaction. The initial reaction is one of shock when the person has difficulty in realising that the death has occurred and may attempt to deny it. This is followed by a period of great unhappiness and sadness and a yearning for the deceased

which may continue for a few weeks. Anorexia, guilt feelings and preoccupation with thoughts of the deceased are also observed during this period. A few weeks after, the final stage of the reaction may take place and this is characterised by acceptance of the fact that the loss is irretrievable, and by re-adjustment to life. Most grief reactions are resolved within a six month period but some may go on for a year or more and take on the features of a depressive illness. Factors which suggest that the death of the sister was an important life event in precipitating the patient's illness is that the sister was of course a first degree relative, with whom she had a close relationship and the observation of the relatives that the patient has never been well since the death of the sister, and is pre-occupied with thoughts of her.

Q3.

Parkinson's disease appears to be related to psychiatric illness in two contexts. Firstly there is the direct relationship, and secondly the indirect relationship related to the effects of drugs used in the treatment of Parkinsonism. Depressed affect has been found in up to 40 per cent of untreated patients with Parkinsonism and the degree of depression is related to the severity of the illness. Dementia is now considered to be a common accompaniment of Parkinson's disease, although it was never commented on by Parkinson in his original description. It is stated by various researchers that between $\frac{1}{5}$ and $\frac{1}{3}$ of patients with Parkinson's disease show signs of cognitive impairment and this is most commonly found in the arteriosclerotic type. The exhibition of L-dopa in the treatment of Parkinsonism, while improving the physical condition, may increase the frequency and aggravate the severity of depression.

Q4.

Although anaemia has some symptoms characteristic of endogenous depression such as tiredness, malaise and apathy and may be an accompaniment of depression due to loss of appetite, there is no substantial evidence that anaemia causes depression. However, there is a need to further elucidate the significance of low levels of haemotinics such as vitamin B12 and folic acid observed in some depressed patients. Appetite disturbance of course could reduce the levels.

Q5.

Psychiatric patients in general are unreliable in taking medication as prescribed. Estimates as low as 40 per cent compliance have been made with psychiatric patients in general and it is likely that due to varying degrees of cognitive impairment and the likelihood of taking many kinds of medication simultaneously, that elderly psychiatric patients have an even lower compliance. Efforts by pharmaceutical firms to ensure that elderly patients receive appropriate medication have centered on providing the total daily medication in one long-lasting package to be taken at night or morning.

Q6.

The 'monoamine hypothesis' proposes that depression is due mainly to a depletion of monoamine neurotransmitters in certain parts of the brain and that mania is associated with an excess of these substances. The neurotransmitters which have received most attention are the catecholamines dopamine and noradrenaline, and serotonin which is an indoleamine. Attempts at verifying this hypothesis have included biochemical examination of the brains of patients who have committed suicide, examination of C.S.F. and urine for the concentration of these substances or of their metabolites and the observation of the effects of the administration of antagonists or precursors on individuals. It appears from post-mortem studies that depression is associated with abnormal brain serotonin turnover. In the C.S.F. and the urine the metabolites of brain serotonin, noradrenaline, and dopamine namely, 5 hydroxyindoleacetic acid (5 H.I.A.A.) 3 methoxy-4-hydroxy-phenylethyleneglycol (M.H.P.G.) and homovanilic acid (HVA) respectively, are measured and some studies suggest abnormal results in depression.

Q7.

The main shortcomings of the 'monoamine hypothesis' are firstly that it is an over simplified view of such a complex psychobiological event as affective illness which may be intimately related to and influenced by personality, social and environmental factors. Secondly although the theory has stimulated research in brain biochemistry it has not superseded more primitive empirical research in providing effective treatment for affective disorders. Thirdly there are considerable methodological problems in measuring accurately the level of monoamines and their metabolites in body fluids and excluding the possibility of error induced by non-central nervous system sources of these substances, and studies on post-mortem brains are open to error by the biochemical changes which take place at the time of death. Fourthly efforts at influencing the course of affective illness by serotonin precursors such as tryptophan, or antagonists such as methysergide, have been generally unsuccessful.

Finally there has also been a marked inconsistency among researchers in this field. More recent commentators on this theory suggest that the theory is inadequate because the affective psychoses are biochemically heterogenous, that reduced serotonin is a constant finding not only in depression but also in those prone to depression, and that the chemical abnormality is to be found in the receptor sites and not at the level of the neurotransmitters. It is likely that the theory will have to be revised considerably in the future.

Q8.

This patient should be admitted to hospital for antidepressant treatment as she is unreliable in taking medication at home. A further trial of tricyclic antidepressants preferably those with little cardio-toxic effects and ideally one that could be taken only once a day should be tried. If she is unresponsive to this then, due to the long ongoing period of depression she has endured, there should be little delay in prescribing E.C.T. After recovery she should continue with antidepressants for approximately six months and she should be followed up at outpatients and should be visited regularly by the community psychiatric nurse to ensure that she complies with medical advice.

Course and management

After a further trial of tetracyclic antidepressants to which the patient failed to respond, she was treated with a course of six E.C.T.'s to which she made a good response. She was discharged from hospital to be supervised by the community psychiatric nurse. She continues to take tetracyclic antidepressants three time daily and is followed up at outpatients.

Further reading

Brown G W, Harris T O, Peto J 1973 Life events and psychiatric disorder II: nature of the causal link, Psych Med 3: 159–176

Eccleston D 1981 Monoamines in depression. Brit J Psychiat 138: 257–258
Eccleston D 1982 The biochemistry of the affective disorders. Brit J Hosp Med 27(6): 627–634

Mindham R H S 1974 Psychiatric aspects of Parkinson's disease. Brit J Hosp Med 2: 411–14

Van Praag H M, Korf J, Lakke J P W F, Schut T 1975 Dopamine metabolism in depressive psychoses and Parkinson's disease. The problem of the specificity of biological variables in behaviour disorders. Psych Med 5: 138–146

CASE 27

A 65-year-old man is admitted to a psychiatric hospital from a casualty department where he had been treated after stabbing himself in the abdomen with a kitchen knife which penetrated only the skin and muscle. He did this he says because 'my stomach is twisted and cramped and my bowels are clogged and nothing can be done for me'. He was born in England, the second eldest of five children of a railway clerk. There is no history of psychiatric illness in the family background. He claims to have had a happy childhood, got on well with his parents and at school and as far as he can tell had no childhood neurotic traits. After leaving school at the age of 14 he worked as a joiner's apprentice for a few weeks, then with a greengrocer and eventually joined the army at the age of 22. He married also at the age of 22 and has one daughter, but was divorced seven years later as his wife 'could not put up with my continual complaints'. He lives alone and is unemployed. During the war he first experienced abdominal pains while in a rifle brigade and spent six weeks in sick bay, and subsequently at regular intervals complained of similar pains and bouts of weakness which remained undiagnosed. He was suspected of malingering, was downgraded and eventually invalided out of the army. He denies that his symptoms were a reaction to the stress of army life, but says he never liked being in the army. The abdominal pains continued but numerous investigations could not detect an organic basis for the symptoms. He smokes about 20 cigarettes daily but drinks very little alcohol, and describes himself as conscientious but sensitive, a very poor mixer with few friends. There is a long psychiatric history dating back to his first admission to a psychiatric hospital in the early 1950's when he was diagnosed as suffering with depression and treated with E.C.T. but with no marked improvement. Over the years he has had about 10 admissions to psychiatric hospitals and has been treated with antidepressants, tranquillisers and E.C.T. but with no marked sustained improvement. He was leucotomised in 1962 but this was also ineffective in relieving his symptoms. For the previous two months his symptoms have increased in severity, but he denies that he is depressed, saying only that he is worried and upset. Three days prior to admission he 'realised that nothing could be done for me', so he decided to kill himself and stabbed himself in his room but called the landlord for help after he did so and was taken to casualty. At interview he is a thin man, looks apprehensive and anxious, he denies feeling depressed, and apart from his apprehensive facies there is no objective evidence of depression. During the interview he continually refers to his abdominal symptoms while his ideas about the state of his stomach and his intestines disclosed in such statements as 'my bowels are rotten, I can't eat, I haven't been to the toilet for days', are bordering on the delusional. There is otherwise no perceptual or cognitive disturbance and he is not suicidal. Physical examination is negative.

Questions

1. What is your formulation on this patient?

2. What is your understanding of the genesis of hypochondriasis?

3. How important as an etiological factor in his illness was this man's army experience?

4. Would you briefly discuss, in the context of psychiatric treatment the following statement, 'Brain surgery should be reserved for brain pathology'?

5. What types of psychosurgery do you know of?

6. How do you distinguish between hysterical and hypochondriacal symptoms?

7. How would you treat this patient?

Answers

Q1.
This man is suffering from a chronic primary monosymptomatic hypochondriacal state. It is described as primary as it does not appear to be associated with another psychiatric condition such as depression, and monosymptomatic because his symptoms have always related to his gastro-intestinal tract. The duration of his symptomatology, his age and the resistence his condition has displayed to treatment suggests that the prognosis is poor.

Q.2
The genesis of hypochondriasis is poorly understood but two related concepts have been proposed, the first is the concept of abnormal illness behaviour and the second is the concept of the interoceptive

set, 'perceptual reactance' or stimulus augumentation. People will respond to a noxious stimulus (interoceptive stimulus) in a continuum of reactions varying between stoical acceptance to hypochondriasis. This reaction is called the perceptual reactance and its nature is determined not only by the constitution of the individual but also by his early learning behaviour and the presence or absence of current psychiatric illness. The ideal response to the noxious stimulus is to behave in a fashion that would attract the attention of the doctor so that the cause or the symptom is removed. However, patients who exhibit abnormal illness behaviour seem to seek ongoing care rather than cure. This ongoing care confirms and reinforces their abnormal reactance to the noxious stimulus and results in hypochondriasis which in this context could be described as learned abnormal illness behaviour.

Q.3.

It is difficult to say precisely how important his army experience was as an etiological factor. It appears that his experience of army life was an unhappy one. His symptoms first appeared while he was a soldier, persisted throughout his service period, he was accused of being a malingerer and was downgraded and eventually discharged. The unpleasant aspect of his army life could have represented a noxious interoceptive stimulus to which he may have responded with a reaction of abnormal illness behaviour and this behaviour would be reinforced as long as he remained in the army. After discharge from the army abnormal illness behaviour may have been his way of dealing with stress, of maintaining his own self-esteem and the esteem of others and may have represented an ongoing effort to validate his symptoms and invalidate the label of a malingerer.

Q4.

Brain surgery in the psychiatric treatment context means psychosurgery and the statement is basically a criticism of psychosurgery. Although psychosurgery has existed as a form of psychiatric treatment since the 1930's it remains the most controversial treatment form in psychiatry. The reasons for the controversy are due primarily to the fact that critics assert that with the vast majority of patients coming for treatment there is no discernible brain pathology which needs surgical intervention, that (at least up to recently) the effects of surgery are irreversible and that the operations are accompanied by a high rate of undesirable psychological side effects such as aggressive psychopathic and impulsive behaviour. With the development of more precise surgical techniques some of the above criticisms are being met. However, a consensus on the type of patient best suited for operation and especially on the type of operation most appropriate, is lacking even amongst the most ardent advocates of treatment, accurate statistics are very difficult to obtain, there are discrepancies in research findings, and there is an obvious need for large studies to elucidate its standing as a treatment form. It is quite possible that for a very small percentage of patients especially those suffering from chronic intractable anxiety, depressive, obsessional or phobic states it may be uniquely indicated. The fact that gross brain pathology is not discernible in the vast majority of patients, does not prove that brain pathology does not exist on the neuronal level. To the degree that it can be consistently shown that surgical interference with certain cerebral pathways has an overall beneficial effect on psychiatric patients then to that degree surgical intervention is valid.

Q5.
The types of psychosurgery could be broadly divided into two. Firstly, there are the older techniques, probably not in use anywhere now. These comprised rather primitive methods for destroying non-specified areas of the frontal lobes. Undesirable psychological effects and post-operative problems were relatively common. The newer techniques are more sophisticated and precise and are dependent on stereotactic instruments. These techniques enable the surgeon, while the head is positioned in a fixed plane, to pin-point the area of the brain in which he wishes to place the lesion, and provide three dimentional maps to facilitate accuracy. Brain scanners and special kinds of X-ray further facilitate such accuracy. The method of destroying brain tissue has evolved, from the surgical knife to such methods as the use of radio frequency waves, radio isotopes, freezing and thermocoagulation. As there appears to be no international consensus as to what are the best techniques and where are the optimum areas of brain to place a lesion for relief of specific problems there is naturally a variety of operations. In general more frontal lobe operations are performed in Britain and these are sometimes combined with cingulotomies and then the whole procedure is defined as a 'limbic leucotomy'. In America cingulotomies and multiple target surgery is more common than in Britain. Psychosurgery has also been advocated in some countries for the treatment of deviant sexual or aggressive and violent behaviour and of course such treatment is ethically controversial. The hypothalamic nuclei appear to be the target areas for such procedures, and ablation of these nuclei have also been performed for the treatment of severe obesity.

Q6.

It can be difficult to distinguish between hysterical and hypochondriacal symptoms as both may present in many forms (and together, e.g. Briquet's syndrome) with symptoms related to such areas as the gastro-intestinal tract and to muscles, joints and bones. The symptoms must be viewed in the setting of the overall presentation, with special reference to age, sex and previous history. Features which may be of help in distinguishing between the two are that hysterical symptoms are more common in females and hypochondriacal symptoms in males, that hysteria is more common in the younger age groups and may be accompanied by more obvious secondary gain, may be more dramatic in presentation, or accompanied by belle indifference and can mimic all other physical diseases, whereas hypochondriasis is more likely to be accompanied by distress and concurrent psychiatric illness, particularly depression.

Q7.

The patient will be difficult to treat successfully because monosymptomatic hypochondriasis is generally resistant to treatment and his symptoms are of long duration. Various types of treatment including simple supportive psychotherapy, behaviour therapy, drugs and psychosurgery have been prescribed but the patient has failed in the past to show any marked response to these. He should in the first instance be admitted for assessment as he appears particularly distressed by his symptoms at present. A long acting I.M. depot preparation, e.g. fluphenazine decanoate may be worthwhile trying and if the acute distress subsides the possibility of discharge could be considered with referral to a day hospital where a nurse therapist could establish a therapeutic relationship with him, give him supportive psycho-therapy and monitor his progress. It is probable that he will fluctuate between good and bad periods and maybe admission to hospital during the bad periods is advisable. There appears to be little alternative to ongoing psychiatric contact either at the medical or para-medical level for this patient.

Course and management

The patient was admitted to hospital and treated with fluphenazine decanoate 40 mg I.M. every two weeks. There was some amelioration of his symptoms and he was discharged to be followed up at outpatients and by a community psychiatric nurse.

Further reading

Bartlett J J, Bridges P, Kelly D 1981 Contemporary indications for psychosurgery. Brit J Psychiat 138: 507–511

Bebbington P E 1976 Monosymptomatic hypochondriasis, abnormal illness behaviour and suicide. Brit J Psychiat 128: 475–478

Bridges P K, Bartlett J J 1977 Psychosurgery: yesterday and today. Brit J Psychiat 131: 249–260

Pilowsky I 1970 Primary and secondary hypochondriasis. Acta Psychiat Scand 46: 273–285

Pilowsky I 1978 A general classification of abnormal illness behaviours. Brit J Med Psychol 51: 131–137

CASE 28

A 67-year-old lady is referred from the surgical department of a general hospital for the treatment of an anxiety state; she was operated on six months previously for peptic ulceration and is physically well. She is the second of four siblings, her father was a farmer. She claims to have had a happy childhood and a good relationship with both parents and there were no childhood neurotic traits such as nocturnal enuresis, school phobia, temper tantrums, or nail biting; as far as she can recall there is no family history of psychiatric illness. After leaving school at 14 she worked on the parents' farm until the age of 18 when she got a job doing domestic work in a hotel and stayed at this type of work for most of her working life and eventually achieved the position of assistant cook in a small hotel. She is heterosexual, had two boyfriends but never married. She does not smoke, drinks very moderately and lives alone in a small flat. Up to the age of 65 she continued to work and did voluntary work in her spare time, she likes reading and has a small circle of friends. All her life she has been a great worrier and says 'I'm inclined to look ahead and expect the worst to happen, I find it hard to relax, especially while lying in bed, the worst fears come to mind'. She has a history of diabetes mellitus of about 20 years duration which has been controlled by diet, and she has had two operations for peptic ulceration, the most recent one six months previously. There is no psychiatric history but she has received diazepam from her family doctor and says this was 'to control my nerves'. At interview she appears to be a rather tense woman who sits very upright in the chair, she is polite and her answers are relevant and to the point. She admits to feeling tense, anxious and worried, but also says that there is no particular problem she is aware of that would justify her anxiety. There is no subjective feeling of depression of mood, no cognitive impairment or psychotic features evident, and she is not suicidal. She does not admit to any disturbance of appetite, but she is inclined to lie awake in bed for a long time at night thinking over the potential problems likely to arise in the future. She is taking diazepam 5 mg t.d.s. but no other medication and she has never abused drugs. She admits that alcohol reduces her tension but she only drinks on special occasions and then very modestly. She says she occasionally experiences palpitations but is otherwise well, and physical examination reveals a pulse rate of 82 per min, slight tremor of the hands, increased reflexes, but otherwise no abnormality and investigations including thyroid function tests are negative.

Questions

1. What is your formulation on this patient?

2. What is your concept of the term psychosomatic illness?

3. Do you know of any interactions between psychological status and diabetes mellitus?

4. As a psychiatrist would you very briefly comment on the following statement 'Anxiety is necessary to keep the cobwebs off the brain'?

5. How would you classify anxiety states?

6. How would you treat this patient?

7. What is the current view on the role of beta-adrenoceptor blocking drugs in the treatment of anxiety states?

Answers

Q1.
This lady is suffering from a chronic anxiety state, with subjective somatic symptoms. Although there is no psychiatric history it is likely that her anxiety is of very long duration and may have been a major factor in producing her condition of peptic ulceration, which could be regarded as a psychosomatic complication of her anxiety state. If her anxiety state can be controlled then of course there should also be less likelihood of further psychosomatic complications. The prospects for full resolution of her state are not good because of the long term duration of her condition and primarily because constitutionally she is a tense apprehensive person.

Q2.
Although the view that some physical diseases have psychological causes has existed from ancient times, the word 'psychosomatic' is relatively recent and has so far defied satisfactory definition. There are a few reasons for this. Clinicians appear to have difficulty in viewing patients in a holistic way, and the tendency has been to keep the psyche and the soma apart. This dualistic approach has militated against clinicians taking the overview of illness and against any concept of psychosomatic illness receiving universal acceptance. It

has also proved difficult to show clearly that psychiatric conditions are directly causative of physical illnesses or indeed antedate the physical illness or are not just associative rather than causative. Conversely many physical illnesses may antedate or precipitate their associated psychiatric illnesses or expose weakness in the personality. There is, however, general agreement that as the brain appears to be the centre of malfunctioning in many psychiatric states, this will be adversely reflected in target areas under neurochemical control. More recent studies of the psychosomatic concept are directed not only at how psychological factors effect the soma but also the effect of personality type on both the incidence and outcome of physical illness. For example there is evidence that the presence of certain abnormal personality characteristics militate against successful surgical intervention for peptic ulceration and survival after myocardial infarction. The psychosomatic concept will only find universal acceptance when it can be validated scientifically; at present an acceptable working definition is the following 'Those conditions where anatomo-pathological or physiopathological changes are evident or where symptoms suggest that such changes occur and in which psychological conditions are held to play an important role in their genesis or aggravation.

Q3.

Diabetes mellitus is not clearly and consistently related to psychological status. Nevertheless there is evidence that emotional factors influence carbohydrate tolerance in diabetes. In stressful situations in particular a psychiatric diabetic patient may over react with increased autonomic activity leading to excessive lipolysis, ketosis and blood glucose shifts. There may also be an increase in maladaptive self management behaviour among psychiatric patients with problems ranging from failure to test urine, to skipping insulin, or over or underdosing. It has also been observed that diabetic children have greater dependency needs, greater anxiety, more hostility and poorer peer relationships than controls, and intelligence may be impaired if the illness starts before the age of five. Arteriopathy in later life, especially in poorly controlled diabetics, may lead to psychiatric complications. There also appears to be a direct relationship between diabetic control in children and improved family relationships. Psychiatric support may influence not only compliance among psychiatric diabetic patients but also the susceptibility of the patient to psychological and biological stress.

Q4.

The axiom that underlies this truism is that a certain amount of anxiety is a pre-requisite to effective functioning and is the driving force behind positive action. In this context anxiety can be viewed alongside other drives such as sex, hunger and thirst. In normal functioning, the feeling of anxiety should be followed and reduced by appropriate behaviour. Each increment of anxiety should be followed by an equal increment in appropriate behaviour and this is normally found up to an optimum level of anxiety associated with advantageous functioning. If this normal optimum level is exceeded for the individual then a catastrophic stage is reached, characterised by disadvantageous functioning. Therefore anxiety as a symptom must always be assessed in the context of its effect on behviour. Conversely the complete absence of anxiety is of course pathological as it is likely to be associated with complete absence of advantageous functioning.

Q5.
There is no clear cut classification of anxiety states due to considerable overlap with depression and to difficulties in assessing the relative importance of such factors as stress, personality and concurrent psychiatric conditions in the etiology of anxiety. There is doubt whether anxiety states exist in pure culture. Although there are objective and subjective somatic disturbances detectable, there are no physiological or biochemical disturbances specific to anxiety. The most practical attempt at classfication at present would appear to be a clinical one. In the clinical setting the description of 'state' and 'trait' is frequently applied to anxiety. 'Trait' anxiety refers to a personality characteristic while 'state' anxiety refers to a situational feeling as when an individual is exposed to a stressful situation such as when facing examinations or going for an operation. 'State' anxiety may be a normal response to a stressful situation, there is also frequently an absence of physiological or behavioural abnormality. Another type of anxiety encountered in practice is that related to a concurrent psychiatric illness to which it may be primary or secondary. Anxiety is further described as diffuse or free floating when unrelated to any particular event and situational when related to a specific event. Anxiety has been further divided into acute or chronic but these terms are usually reserved for patients whose anxiety does not appear to be related to concurrent psychiatric illness. The acute anxiety states are characterised by a short history of illness and good response to treatment and the chronic anxiety states by a long history with poor response to treatment.

Q6.
This patient can be treated as an outpatient. She should continue

to take diazepam 5 mg t.d.s. and since palpitations, tachycardia and tremor appear to be prominent a beta-adrenoceptor blocking drug such as propranolol could also be prescribed. She should be followed up at outpatients to observe the effects of medication and, as there may be some social isolation present, attendance at a day centre or day hospital a few days weekly could be considered. Some supportive psychotherapy might be beneficial.

Q7.

The role of beta-adrenoceptor blocking drugs in the treatment of anxiety states has not yet been clarified. It has been established that they are superior to placebo in treatment but how they compare in efficacy with other anxiety reducing drugs has not been fully resolved. They have their greatest effect on somatic symptoms of anxiety and this is to be expected from their physiological function. Organs or organ systems subjected to beta-adrenergic stimulation will be most influenced by blockade, and therefore the tremor and tachycardia of anxiety will be reduced, and anxious patients subjectively aware of these abnormalities will benefit most. Patients with symptoms of nausea, muscle tension and sweating which are not produced by beta-adrenergic stimulation are unlikely to show comparable improvement.

Course and management

The patient improved with diazepam 5 mg t.d.s. and a tricyclic antidepressant attends a day centre two days weekly, and is followed up at outpatients regularly.

Further reading

Bennet G 1976 Whole-person medicine and psychiatry for medical students. Lancet 1: 623–626

Pond D A 1978 Is the term 'psychosomatic' still of any value. In: Gaind R N, Hudson B L (eds) Current themes in psychiatry, Macmillan Press Ltd, London and Basingstoke

Tyrer P 1982 Anxiety. Brit J Hosp Med 27(2): 109–116

Wilkinson D G 1981 Psychiatric aspects of diabetes mellitus. Brit J Psychiat 138: 1–9

Zealley A K 1978 Psychiatry in medical practice. In: Forrest A D, Affleck J W, Zealley K C (eds) Companion to psychiatric studies, 2nd edn, Churchill Livingstone, Edinburgh, London.

CASE 29

A 74-year-old woman is seen on a domiciliary consultation at the request of her general practitioner who describes her as depressed, agitated and washing her hands so frequently that the skin is cracked and broken. She is a widow, lives alone in a first floor flat and has two daughters both married. Her father was a carpenter, there were five other siblings in the family and she was the second child. There is no history of psychiatric illness in the family background, and she had a happy childhood and as far as she can recall there is no history of childhood neurotic traits. At the age of 14 she left school and worked in a printer's office as a semi-skilled clerk until she married at the age of 25. The husband worked as a messenger for a banking firm and it was a happy marriage, and he died four years previously. There is no previous psychiatric history and she has been well medically, but three months previously she had an operation for diverticulitis and now has a permanent colostomy. She describes herself as a quiet conscientious person with few friends, she is described by one of her children as always 'very neat and fastidious and inclined to be a bit of a worrier'. She doesn't smoke and drinks very modestly on special occasions. The patient was well up to about six weeks previously when she became very worried about the functioning of the colostomy, began changing the bag more often than was necessary and could not keep her mind off its functioning. After each change of bag she began washing her hands for long periods and scrubbed them vigorously with a hard brush. After a time she felt compelled to wash her hands even though she had not recently changed the bag. She became very concerned about cleanliness and tidiness, refused to touch newspapers because she might get contaminated and also became increasingly agitated and restless, her appetite deteriorated, she lost half a stone in weight, her sleep was disturbed and she awoke in the early hours of the morning and had difficulty in getting off to sleep. At interview she is a small thin lady with an anxious apprehensive facies, she is neatly dressed and the flat is immaculately clean and well furnished, but she describes it as a 'rubbish tip'. It is difficult to steer the conversation away from the subject of the colostomy. One of the children says that she has never really accepted the colostomy as permanent but regards it 'more as a wound that will eventually heal'. There is no cognitive impairment and there are no psychotic features evident. She admits to feeling depressed, mainly because of the worry she is giving her children but she denies suicidal feelings. At times she gets into a panic and feels 'I'm going to die', she goes out and knocks on the neighbours' doors irrespective of time, when these feelings come over her: she has only experienced these attacks since she started 'worrying about the colostomy'.

Questions

1. What is your formulation on this patient?

2. What is the relationship between obsessional rumination and ritualistic behaviour?

3. What do you understand by the term 'panic attacks'?

4. As a liaison psychiatrist would you briefly comment on the Hippocratic statement, 'It is not enough for us to do what we can do, the patient and his environment and external conditions must contribute to achieve the cure'?

5. How typical of depression is this woman's disorder of sleep?

6. Briefly do you know of any evidence of endocrine dysfunction in affective disorders?

7. What is the dexamethasone suppression test?

8. How would you treat this patient?

Answers

Q1.

This woman is suffering from depression with endogenous features and a superimposed obsessive compulsive symptom complex. There are disturbances in appetite and secondary weight loss, disturbances in sleep and concentration. She has marked obsessive ruminative features centred on the functioning of her colostomy and also exhibits compulsive hand washing, and experiences panic attacks. The psychological trauma presented by the colostomy to a personality described as always 'very neat and fastidious' may have been the major factor in precipitating her psychiatric condition, as her problem seems to date from shortly after she had the operation and there is no psychiatric history.

Q2.

There are two common current hypotheses on this relationship. The first states that ruminations are noxious stimuli which arise in the setting of altered mood states most commonly depression of mood. Obsessionals are particularly sensitive to these stimuli and are unable to deal with them or dismiss them by any mental mechanism. Their persistence results in increased depression of mood and anxiety and this can only be reduced by repetitive or ritualistic behaviour. The relief gained by the ritual positively re-inforces both the occurrence of the rumination and the ritual. On this hypothesis anxiety and depression would appear to be the major driving force in the genesis of both. A second hypothesis proposes the ruminations and rituals result from a disorder of the arousal system so that incoming stimuli of minor noxious import are viewed as of major importance and result in major defensive reactions. The resultant obsessional and ritualistic reaction is then viewed as a defence mechanism, and the ritual may have a symbolic character, such as washing of hands if the ruminative thought content is of contamination or guilt.

Q3.

A severe unmanageable bout of anxiety precipitated by a situation, an event or an object is considered to be the important underlying factor in the genesis of a panic attack. Panic attacks may therefore be experienced in those psychiatric states in which anxiety is a common component such as obsessional compulsive neurosis, phobic states, and, of course, mixed anxiety and depressive states. In the obsessional state the panic attack may occur when the anxiety overwhelms the individual's method of coping with it, for example when his repetitive or ritualistic behaviour no longer compensates. The agoraphobic or the claustrophobic may experience it when the anxiety stimulated by the environment becomes unmanageable. Panic attacks are almost always accompanied by marked somatic sensations and sometimes a feeling that death or dissolution is imminent and there may be marked over activity of the autonomic nervous system. There is usually an effort at flight or removal of the anxiety provoking stimulus and frequently the presence or help of others is sought, and these manoeuvres limit the duration of the attack. Treatment of panic attacks will be directed at the related concurrent psychiatric state, and may involve physical, psychotherapeutic or behavioural techniques singly or in combination.

Q4.

From the psychiatric viewpoint this statement could be viewed as a plea for a holistic approach to treatment, with attention to the psyche as well as the soma. This would not necessitate psychiatric involvement with all physical illness, indeed, that would be both impractical and undesirable. What is desirable, however, is that physicians should be more aware of the psychological dimension of physical illness and how it may effect treatment and outcome. There is also a need for more liaison psychiatry with more active participation by the psychiatrist in the therapeutic team, for example in the treatment of patients with difficult chronic and painful conditions and in the assessment and preparation of patients about to undergo major surgical procedures such as transplants or amputations. These patients may have to undergo considerable psychological re-adjustment in coping with their stressful conditions and altered body image.

Q5.

Depression is the most common psychiatric illness associated with a disorder of sleep. In the endogenous type of depression early morning waking with difficulty in getting back to sleep is the commonly described type of disturbance, and this is what this patient complains of, while difficulty in getting off to sleep is more characteristic of reactive depression. However, there are diagreements on the validity of this distinction, as descriptions of sleep patterns based solely on patients' reports are often unreliable. Polygraphic and E.E.G. monitoring, however, has shown that depressives in general take longer to get off to sleep, sleep less, have more wakefulness, than controls, and further studies have shown that endogenous depressives, have less total sleep, stage four and R.E.M. sleep than neurotic depressives, though initial or late insomnia patterns have not been established. There are also different research findings on the pattern of R.E.M. sleep in depressives, with results suggesting decreased, increased and normal patterns. Research into sleep disturbance in depression, like many aspects of research in depression is complicated by difficulties in ensuring that the populations studied are really comparable.

Q6.

There is considerable evidence of endocrine dysfunction in affective disorders accumulated from observation of mood disturbance in endocrinological disorders and tests of endocrine function in affective disorders. It is well established that mood changes frequently occur in Addison's disease, Cushing's syndrome and in association with steroid medication. It is also known that cortisol production levels are high in depressives and fall to normal after treatment. Corticotrophin releasing hormone is released from the hypothalamus by lysine vasopressin, which leads to an increased secretion of A.C.T.H. and raised plasma cortisol levels. In some depressed patients this response to lysine vasopressin is not observed. Insulin induced hypoglycaemia is a stimulation test of hypothalamic-pituitary-adrenal *H.P.A.* function and results normally in a rise in plasma cortisol but depressed patients, especially those already with an increased cortisol production rate, appear to be resistant to this stimulation test. Patients with depression also have a greater number of cortisol secretory episodes than controls, and have episodes during the late evening and early morning when normal subjects do not. It is thought that abnormalities of H.P.A. function observed in endogenous depression is not just a stress response but is a phenomenon of equal biological significance to disorders of sleep, appetite, and mood, observed in this condition. Further it should be noted that the pattern of H.P.A. abnormality in depression has many similarities to that observed in diencephalic Cushing's disease, and that some commentators on depression have suggested that the hypothalamus may be the primary centre of malfunction. It has also been observed that the growth hormone response to L-Dopa, apomorphine and hypoglycaemia is impaired in depression. In bipolar manic depressive psychosis it has been postulated that there is a primary defect in the renin system. There is evidence that there is a high resting renin activity and a blunted renin response to Aldosterone production rates. Hypothalamic releasing hormones have important behavioural actions and are considered to be of increasing significance to neuropsychiatry. It is thought by some that the study of these hormones will displace that of the monoamines as the main interest of neuropsychiatric research.

Q7.

The dexamethasone suppression test is based on the observation that there is a diurnal variation in the secretion of cortisol. Dexamethasone given to controls at midnight suppresses the plasma cortisol levels for 24 hours by feedback suppression of A.C.T.H. It has been observed that people with impaired suppression have symptoms patterns suggestive of endogenous depression. No abnormalities were noticed in reactive depression, and so far no abnormalities are noted in hypomania. The test is not established as a clinical diagnostic tool because some researchers have failed to find abnormalities of suppression and because of difficulties in administering the test adequately, which entails taking blood samples about every half hour.

Q8.

As there is such a pronounced depressive component in this woman's case it would be well worthwhile seeing how she would respond to a course of tricyclic antidepressants over a three or four week period. Clomipramine which is reputed to be effective in controlling obsessive compulsive features in the presence of depression could be tried at a dose ranging from 50 to 100 mg t.d.s. This could be tried on an outpatient basis. If panic attacks become severe and frequent or suicide becomes a distinct possibility then admission to hospital may be necessary and if there is failure to respond to antidepressants then a course of E.C.T. could be considered. Supportive psychotherapy aimed at getting the patient to accept the unavoidable necessity of living with the colostomy and training on daily management of it will also probably be indicated. When discharged from hospital attendance at a day centre may help to fill the social vacuum in her life style and reduce the likelihood of morbid ruminations.

Course and management

The patient failed to respond to antidepressants and was admitted to hospital after three weeks. After two more weeks she had a course of six E.C.T.'s and there was considerable improvement in her affect, her obsessive compulsive features become less serious and she had no further panic attacks. She was discharged to attend a day centre and continues to take tricyclic antidepressants and is followed up at outpatients. The prognosis is reasonable.

Further reading

Beaumont P J V 1979 The endocrinology of psychiatry. In: Granville Grossman K (ed) Recent advances in clinical psychiatry 3, Churchill Livingstone, Edinburgh, London

Gomez J 1981 Liason psychiatry. Brit J Hosp Med 26(3): 242–250

LLoyd G G 1977 Psychological reactions to physical illness. Brit J Hosp Med 18: 352–59

Marks I M, Stern R S, Mawson D, Cobb J, McDonald R 1980 Clomipramine and exposure for obsessive compulsive rituals 1 Brit J Psychiat 136: 1–25

Millar H R 1981 Psychiatric morbidity in elderly surgical patients. Brit J Psychiat 138: 17–20

CASE 30

A 17-year-old male presents in psychiatric outpatients accompanied by his parents and a social worker. The parents complain that 'he is uncontrollable at home, terrorises us by throwing knives and assaulting us'. The mother and her sister have a history of epilepsy but there is no psychiatric history in the family background and the marriage is reasonably successful, the patient is the sixth of seven siblings and the husband is a long distance lorry driver. The patient's birth weight was five and a half pounds and the pregnancy although going to full term normal delivery was complicated by toxaemia. As a child he suffered from measles, varicella and pertussis. For the first two and a half years the child's development was normal, but at the age of two and a half he had a major epileptic seizure. He continued to have seizures at varying intervals throughout childhood, especially at night. He was also described as having 'myoclonic attacks' as a child. At the age of five his I.Q. on the Terman-Merrill Scale was 88, and he started to abscond from home, frequently got lost and had to wear an identity disc. Up to the age of seven he was bed wetting, also showed temper tantrums if he was frustrated in his wishes and at the age of eight he was admitted to a residential school for epileptics. An E.E.G. at this time showed considerable abnormality particularly on the left side, but investigations showed no focal organic lesion. A social report says that the parents live in a low rent council house in a run down area. The husband's job necessitates him leaving home at 5:30 a.m. and not returning until after 5 p.m., sometimes later if the opportunity to work overtime arose. Sometimes he would be absent from the home for days on long distance trips and was not of course able to give support to his wife in coping with the child. The mother-in-law gave very practical and emotional support in dealing with the child's behaviour disturbances. Overall the parents' attitude to the child was one of over-protection characterised by the mother's desire to have him in sight always in case he had a fit. She would not allow him to play outside with his siblings for the same reason and he was not disciplined or made to face the consequences of his action like the others. The parents also gave him gifts in the hope that this would keep him happy and he would not misbehave, but he led his mother a 'merry dance' when he escaped from the home. She would chase after him, become very angry with him and start to shout and swear, and he would respond in a similar fashion. Eventually they lost their control over him completely and he was admitted to a residential school for epileptics at the age of eight. He remained there for eight years and his behaviour stabilised and then he started living at home again and attending an adult training centre. Further I.Q. tests showed his overall score as 84. Within one year the parents were in great difficulties with him again, his behaviour had become unpredictable and aggressive and he was now physically violent to the parents and refused to attend the training centre. He continued to have major fits, there was difficulty in getting him to take his medication and he began to drink tea in excessive quantities and started bedwetting. This behaviour has been present for about two months. At interview the patient is very slow in responding to questioning and is incapable of giving an account of himself, he does not appear depressed and there are no psychotic features present. Physical examination is negative. The history is obtained from the parents and the social worker. He is receiving the following medication:- phenytoin 100 mg a.m., 150 mg nocte, primidone 250 mg a.m., 250 mg at 3 p.m. and 250 mg nocte, carbamazepine 400 mg a.m., 200 mg 2 p.m., 400 mg nocte, imipramine 25 mg a.m., 25 mg midday, 50 mg nocte.

QUESTIONS

1. What is your formulation on this patient?

2. How would you investigate this youth?

3. What comments would you make on his medication?

4. What factors precipitate fits?

5. What do you understand of the emotional difficulties of an adolescent mentally handicapped person?

6. What services exist to help a mentally handicapped adolescent and his parents?

7. How would you manage this patient?

Answers

Q1.
This patient is an epileptic educationally subnormal adolescent youth who presents with a behaviour disorder characterised by aggressive

and violent behaviour directed mainly against his parents. While in a structured environment in residential care his behaviour was generally good. It is probable that he misses this environment, since his discharge home and finds it difficult to compete in a large family setting, gets frustrated and this frustration expresses itself in violent and maladaptive behaviour.

Q2.
The first line of investigation is to make sure his general health is good. A general physical examination supported by full blood count, blood sugar, E.S.R. electrolytes, calcium and urea estimations, liver function tests, urinalysis and chest film are important. A neurological examination should exclude deterioration within the nervous system. Drug levels should be estimated at six monthly intervals and because he is receiving anticonvulsants a folic acid estimation done. An important part of the investigation is to observe his behaviour and response to a new environment. This should not be rushed. Help from other colleagues, nurses, trainers and therapists (art, music, drama and occupational) should be obtained. If a skull radiograph, electroencephalograph and brain scan have not been done these should be considered. A record of the frequency of fits should be kept and descriptions of seizures made. One should keep in touch with the family, preferably personally, but also through the services of a social worker. Reports from the managers of the training centre and club leader should be obtained if appropriate. Attitudes between patient, parents and other members of the family should be studied.

Q3.
The programme of medication is too complicated and needs simplifying. Mentally handicapped people, their families and community care staff cannot maintain complicated programmes. Such regimens also interfere with the social life of the patient. The prescribing doctor should take cognisance of the half-life of drugs he prescribes and this should guide him according to the frequency with which a drug is given. The half-lives of the drugs in this case are: carbamazepine 8 to 46 hours, primidone 3 to 12 hours, phenytoin 10 to 42 hours, imipramine 8 to 16 hours. On this basis of their half-lives these drugs need only be given twice daily. It is also very important to try and control epilepsy with one drug alone, especially in subnormal patients who may confuse medication. Imipramine is probably not indicated with this patient.

Q4.

The factors which may precipitate fits can be grouped as follows:-physical factors; light, especially flickering light, e.g. sunlight shining through trees into a moving vehicle, bright light reflecting off rippling water, T.V. screen, fireworks, discos. Noise, if sudden and loud, and music, can precipitate fits in the susceptible. Temperature changes either of body temperature or extremes of environmental temperature are potential hazards as is head injury. Emotional causes such as excitement, anxiety, fear or startle, and insomnia leading to fatigue may do so. Also biochemical changes, including hypoglycaemia, hypocalcaemia, hyponatraemia and water retention are important. Drugs, such as phenothiazines and tricyclics may exacerbate fits. In some females, fits are more frequent premenstrually.

Q5.

Subnormal adolescents feel the same impact of physiological and emotional changes which affect normal children. However, the matter is complicated by the difficulty of being accepted as adults. Behaviour which is tolerable as children becomes unacceptable as adults. Furthermore, adolescent handicapped people are frequently lonely because companionship of contemporaries is difficult to find and sustain. Deprivations lead to insecurity. Difficult behaviours are adopted as a means of solving emotional conflicts. Antisocial behaviour is frequent; in males, aggression, thieving, exposure, fetishes, micturition in public and absconding are common. In girls, fear of pregnancy leads to deprivation of opportunity to mix and become independent. Both sexes have difficulties in maintaining regular employment. The less severely handicapped adolescent is likely to have complications of a more serious and prolonged nature than those who are more severely affected. If he is living at home jealousies occur because he feels he cannot compete with his normal brothers and sisters, either in school (homework), or at work or in having friends of the opposite sex. Management is, therefore, complicated by family and environmental matters. It is common for the adolescent to develop anxieties (disturbances of appetite, communication difficulty, insomnia, polydypsia, nightmares and night terrors, enuresis and soiling) and depression.

Q6.

Most adolescents can be helped if they are living at home through a variety of people, community services and voluntary agencies.

These include the community nurse, (this person has mental handicap training as well as special training in community work) and the social worker. In this patient's case a programme had been worked out along the following lines: the patient had been placed in a residential training unit for epileptics and the unit and social worker worked out a regime in which it was hoped that the patient would learn to take responsibility for his behaviour and face the consequences. The social worker counselled the parents on their relationship with the patient to enable them to achieve the same end and the unit liaises with the social worker over the patient's contact with his parents, i.e. what happens at visits and parental contact with the unit concerning the demands that the patient makes to them on the telephone. Help can also be obtained from the general practitioner, the manager and staff of the Adult Training Centre (ATC.), the co-ordinator of residential care, (a social services appointment who organises residential care, hostel, boarding out), the disablement resettlement officer (DRO), the community assessment and treatment team or community mental handicap team (these are multidisciplinary teams consisting of psychiatrist, community nurse, social worker, psychologist, other therapists (occupational, physiotherapist, speech therapist, music, drama and art). Club activities are organised either by social services or voluntary organisations such as Gateway Clubs or Mencap. Holiday schemes usually run by social services and voluntary organisations are available. Help with extra recreational activities can be obtained through adventure playgrounds sponsored by the National Playing Fields Association and Play for the Handicapped, and sporting activities are organised through social services or charities such as Special Olympics, United Kingdom. A programme of adult and further education is available through local Education Authorities. With regard to sex counselling, parents get a great deal of support either from their local Parent Society or through Mencap. Parent's workshops are a means of counselling and general support — these are usually organised by statutory bodies. If an adolescent is judged to have a medical problem such as anxiety or depression then appropriate medication will be needed. Epilepsy will need specific drug therapy.

Q7.
It is probably advisable in the first instance to readmit this patient to the residential home for the mentally subnormal epileptic. This will give an opportunity to medical and paramedical personnel to investigate the home situation and try and identify stressful aspects

for the patient living at home. Admission to residential care will also alleviate the stress in the overburdened parents and afford an opportunity for re-assessing the patient medically and psychologically. It may be possible to reduce the variety of medication he is receiving. When the behaviour pattern improves trial leave periods at home should be initiated before deciding on final discharge. Attendance at an adult sheltered training centre should again be tried and he should be followed up at outpatients.

Course and management

The patient was again admitted to a residential home for epileptics for further assessment. His behaviour improved considerably in the structured environment of the home. Imipramine and carbamazepine were omitted and he was treated with one anticonvulsant. It was planned to allow him home on trial leave and attend a day centre for occupational therapy and observation.

Further reading

Department of health and social security 1980 Mental handicap progress, problems and priorities. A review of mental handicap services in England since the 1971 White Paper 'Better services for the mentally handicapped'.

National development group for the mentally handicapped 1979 Report: Creating a learning environment. In: Helping mentally handicapped people in hospital, Department of health and social security publication, HMSO, London ch 5, ch 6

Kirman B H 1980 Reading about mental handicap. Brit J Psychiat 137: 491–493

Kotsopoulos S, Maiathia P 1980 Worries of parents regarding the future of their mentally retarded adolescent children. Int J Soc Psychiat 26(1): 53–57

Shorvon S D, Chadwick D, Galbraith S W, Reynolds E H 1978 One drug for epilepsy. Brit Med J 1: 474–476

CASE 31

A patient who has spent a lifetime in long-stay care in a hospital for the mentally handicapped is described. She suffers from mental handicap (severe subnormality) having an I.Q. of 40, was born in 1909 to a mother who was mentally handicapped, and from the age of three, together with her family, moved in and out of work-houses and subsequently various institutions. She has an older sister who is also mentally handicapped. She finally moved into long-stay care at the age of 15 years, at which time she was unable to reply to simple questions and could not repeat numbers or sentences of three or four words, did not know her alphabet and was assessed as having a mental age of a child of three years and therefore unable to take proper care of herself. It was observed that she was unable either to dress or wash herself properly and could not perform any domestic duties, and she often laughed and giggled fatuously. Articulation was poor and when ever spoken to she could give no account of herself. Emotional control was frequently disturbed, she would cry loudly, and frequently hid herself away in corners and was terrified and resistive to physical contact when she had a medical or dental examination. Sometimes she could be quarrelsome and impulsively violent, striking out at other patients. At 43-years she did not know her age and could not count her fingers. She said cows and horses had five legs and could not tell which was the bigger, a hen's egg or an orange. She was babyish in manner having a fixed grin and sucked her fingers repeatedly, and had practically no reasoning powers or judgement and had to be constantly shepherded and supervised in her toilet. Capable of only the simplest repetitive forms of occupation she remains quite lost and helpless away from the familiar environment of the ward. Physically, she is only 145 cm in stature with a weight of 50.8 kg. There are no physical deformities. Menstruation had been regular but ceased at 40 years. A mild left hemiparesis developed at 57 years but this improved gradually. She is physically well and investigations which have included chromosomal, haematological and biochemical tests are negative. There is no evidence of phenylketonuria.

Questions

1. What is your formulation on this case?

2. What do you understand by the term 'subcultural' mental handicap?

3. Would you briefly classify the causes of mental handicap?

4. What is the likelihood that this patient's mother had phenyl-ketonuria?

5. Very briefly give some broad guide lines on the risks mentally handicapped parents present in reproducing and rearing children.

6. Are the mentally handicapped particularly vulnerable to psychiatric illness?

7. Is there any way of preventing or ameliorating subcultural mental handicap?

Answers

Q1.

This patient is a severely subnormal 71-year-old woman, who has spent most of her life in institutions and is grossly institutionalised. There is no obvious cause for her mental subnormality nor does it fit into any particular type of syndrome. She comes from a family background with two members who have been described as subnormal and maybe subcultural subnormality would be the most appropriate diagnosis for this patient, although many facts about the patient's early life are unknown. It is most likely that she will need on-going care and supervision in a sheltered environment.

Q2.

Mental handicap can be broadly divided into a pathological type which, in current thinking, includes all conditions with known medical causes and a subcultural type which is applied to those mentally handicapped without a definable pathological cause. People in the subcultural category are usually found in the less severe and uncomplicated forms of mental handicap. Normal biological variation, as indicated in the Gaussian curve of population distribution has been used to explain the existence of this group. Although this patient would appear to be in the subcultural group, there may be genetic implications, suggested by the family history and in many instances categorisation is often compounded by maternal deprivation and poor social environment, as in this case.

Q3.

The cause of mental handicap is not always clear; however a cause may be found under one of the following headings:-

(a) Genetic — these will include disorders of protein, carbohydrate or fat metabolism, e.g. histidinemia, homocystinuria, maple syrup urine disease, phenylketonuria, galactosemia and the cerebral lipidoses, leucodystrophies, mucopolysaccharidoses, cranial anomalies (primary microcephaly, craniostenosis and congenital hydrocephalus), congenital ectodermoses (tuberous sclerosis, neurofibromatosis, cerebral angiomatosis), chromosomal abnormalities (Down's syndrome, Klinefelter's syndrome, triple X syndrome, hermaphroditism, cri du chat syndrome, trisomies D and E, and others).

(b) Prenatal — these will include maternal and foetal infections (syphilis, rubella, toxoplasmosis, cytomegalic inclusion disease), foetal irradiation, kernicterus (bilirubin encephalopathy), Cretinism, prenatal unknown or indefinite causes associated with placental abnormality, toxaemia of pregnancy, prematurity, maternal medication, poisoning, nutritional deficiency, infection or trauma.

(c) Perinatal — these will include birth injuries, infection, cerebral trauma, haemorrhage, anoxia, hypoglycaemia.

(d) Postnatal — these will include cerebral infections (meningitis, encephalitis, abscess), cerebral trauma, including non-accidental injury, poisoning (lead, carbon monoxide and others), cerebrovascular accidents, occlusion and haemorrhage from congenital defects, deficiency diseases or unknown causes, postimmunization encephalopathy (pertussis, smallpox, rabies and others).

Q4.

The question of 'unclassified' mental retardation does not totally exclude the possibility of biochemical insult having occurred to the developing brain. Such insults may adversely effect the vigorous neuronal multiplication in the foetus. It is known that the foetal brain is vulnerable to damage by excess phenylalanine. Maternal phenylketonuria can be a cause of mental retardation in children without the metabolic defect. The risk to the unborn child is related to the level of phenylalanine in the mother's blood, high levels (above 20 mg/100 ml) carry more risk than low ones (below 20 mg/100 ml). In the case presented the patient does not have phenylketonuria. Unfortunately it is not possible to test the mother for this condition. However, since the mother and two of her children are mentally handicapped the circumstances are suspicious. The patient would be heterozygous for the genetic fault.

Q5.

Sex education and opportunities for mentally handicapped people to have sexual experiences frequently pose the question of risks of them producing mentally handicapped children and of their ability to rear children. There is no precise information on this matter but certain broad guidelines can be considered:-

a. If the mental handicap of the parent(s) is due to acquired pathological conditions other than those linked with hereditary causes then it would be reasonable to assume that a genetically healthy child could be conceived.

b. If either parent carries a recessively inherited disease then children would be heterozygous for that condition. Should prospective parents have receissive disorders the risks to offspring becomes complicated. If they have the same disease then all offspring will have the disease; if their diseases are different the offspring will be heterozygotes for two conditions but could be mentally normal.

c. Dominantly inherited conditions in a parent will carry 50/50 chance of children inheriting the disease.

d. In the case of Down's syndrome females with this should produce normal and trisomic gametes in equal numbers which when fertilised should result in normal and trisomic zygotes in the proportion of 1:1.

e. Disturbed foetal environment is likely to occur in women with abnormal metabolic states, e.g. phenylketonuria, thereby putting development of the foetal brain at risk.

f. In the event of a child being born to mentally handicapped parents there will be the question of management and of healthy child-rearing. This is not necessarily a gloomy outlook but would involve considerable aid from health and social services. Alternative forms of care for the child would be adoption and fostering. It may also have to be considered, that battering parents are frequently found to be in the modest or low intelligence range, and their violence may be indicative of their frustration at not being able to cope.

Q6.

Mentally handicapped people are particularly vulnerable to psychiatric illness. This is thought to be due to brain pathology and the adverse effects of social rejection, family stress and educational failure. Estimates varying from 40 per cent to 60 per cent prevalence for psychiatric disorder among mentally handicapped children contrasts starkly with a 6 per cent prevalence among children in general in Britain. The main disorders encountered are early childhood autism, hyperkinetic symptoms, affective disorders and schizophrenia. There are difficulties in diagnosis because of incomplete development of language, poor communication and ritualistic behaviour which may not be of psychiatric origin. The presence of psychiatric illness is frequently the deciding factor on whether a person lives in the community or in an institution.

Q7.

Subcultural mental handicap can be prevented to a degree or ameliorated by the process of modelling. Children at risk lack emotional and intellectual stimulation because the parents are poorly endowed intellectually or retarded. During the very early years of life such children can be provided with structured nursery and pre-school experiences. Also parents at risk of rearing such children may be introduced to educational programmes and learn by the process of modelling, that is the parent (or the child) is taught to imitate the actions of the teacher.

Course and management

There is no specific treatment other than caring for her physical, emotional and social needs and creating the optimum life style suitable for her within the hospital setting.

Further reading

Clarke A M, Clarke A D B 1974 Mental deficiency, the changing outlook, Methuen, London

Cowie V 1980 Injury and insult — considerations of the neuropathological etiology of mental subnormality. Brit J Psychiat 187: 305–312

Lewis D 1933 Types of mental deficiency and their social significance. J Ment Sci 79: 298–294

Mabry C C, Denniston J C, Nelson T L, Son C D 1963 Maternal phenylketonuria: a cause of mental retardation in children without the metabolic effect. New Eng Med J 269: 1404

Reid A H 1982 The psychiatry of mental handicap, Blackwell Scientific Publications, Oxford

Richards B W 1974 Case and kindred in mental deficiency. Brit J Psychiat 125: 547–552

CASE 32

A lady of 39-years is presented at a psychiatric case conference, for retrospective review of her diagnosis. She is the eldest of three children and the parents are both alive. The father is a successful business man and the mother has a history of depression, having been treated on two occasions in hospital. There is no other history of psychiatric illness in the family background. She had a reasonably happy childhood, used to bite her nails and was enuretic up to the age of seven. She was near the top of the class scholastically and left school after doing 'O' levels at the age of 17, and did a shorthand and typing course and got a job as a secretary. Most of her life she has worked as a secretary but for a few years she worked as a public relations officer for a charitable organisation. She is heterosexual and had a few relationships with men, one of six years duration but she never married because the man she wished to marry she describes as having 'let her down'. She describes herself as a friendly energetic person who drinks and smokes moderately, and likes to 'put everything I've got into a job, I'm a workaholic'. Her interests are mainly in swimming and tennis and she has been physically well all her life. She was first admitted to a psychiatric hospital at the age of 21 after taking an overdose of drugs while depressed, and relates this depression to the tragic death of a young friend six weeks previously. She was diagnosed as suffering with endogenous depression with loss of appetite, sleep disturbance and anergia, and was treated with E.C.T. After five weeks she was discharged much improved. She continued to take tricyclic antidepressants and remained well for about three years when she again suffered with depression, lost her appetite and two stone in weight. She also experienced one bout of hearing voices, they came from within her head, spoke to her rather than about her and she never experienced this before or after. At the time she was fully awake and had not abused drugs. On this occasion she was admitted to hospital and schizophrenia was considered to be the likely diagnosis. Again she responded to a course of six E.C.T.'s and was well for about a year and a half until she was apprehended for shoplifting and taking the car of a friend without his permission. On this occasion she was regarded by the general practitioner as depressed and was admitted to hospital. She slashed her wrists while in hospital and was regarded as suffering from endogenous depression in the setting of a vulnerable personality with psychopathic traits. There were no psychotic features evident. She was treated with tricyclic antidepressants and discharged after four weeks and has remained well for the last thirteen years, has held down a responsible secretarial position and is socially active. At interview the patient is symptom free psychiatrically and appears quite normal mentally.

Questions

1. In the light of hindsight attempt a formulation on this patient.

2. Would you describe this patient's auditory experience as a pseudo-hallucination?

3. How predictive of adult psychiatric disturbance at the time of occurrence was this woman's childhood neurotic traits of nail biting and enuresis?

4. How reliable are psychiatric diagnoses?

5. Very briefly discuss the views of Thomas S. Szasz on psychiatric diagnoses.

6. Apart from those of Schneider what other diagnostic criteria of schizophrenia are you aware of?

7. What do you know of the United States — United Kingdom diagnostic project?

8. What is the prognosis for this woman?

Answers

Q1.

It is quite probable that this patient was not suffering with schizophrenia, certainly not process schizophrenia, and she only experienced one episode of auditory hallucinations, these hallucinations not having the Schneiderian characteristics of discussing the patient in the third person, repeating the patient's thoughts out loud or commenting on the patient's behaviour. What is more probable is that the patient had a depressive illness with endogenous features such as disturbance of appetite, sleep and drive, and this responded to tricyclic antidepressants and E.C.T. Her personality could probably have been more accurately described as maturing rather than vulnerable or psychopathic as she now appears to be a very well adjusted personality.

Q2.

This patient's auditory experience could probably be described as a pseudo-hallucination. She was fully conscious at the time and not under the influence of drugs. She described the voice as coming from within her head, this being typical of pseudo-hallucinations, which in common terminology have been described as the voice of the mind or the voice of conscience and as the patient was depressed at the time she may have been particularly pensive or withdrawn. Pseudo-hallucinations may coexist with or progress to true hallucinations but in isolation pseudo-hallucinations may not be of morbid portent.

Q3.

At the time it was probably not very predictive. It has been accepted for many years that there is a strong association between childhood neurotic traits and adult psychiatric illness especially adult neurosis, and the format for psychiatric case taking always includes questions to elicit whether childhood neurotic traits existed. Current consensus opinion, however, maintains that while childhood neurosis and neurotic traits carry an increased risk of adult neurosis, this risk is far less than was previously believed. It is estimated that only 3–4 per cent of children with neurosis who attend clinics become adult attenders.

Q4.

It is probably still true that in clinical practice psychiatric diagnoses are unreliable. There are many factors contributing to their unreliability. Firstly, there are the subjective biases of the psychiatrists, which may have been exacerbated by training in particular schools, or by espousal of particular orientations. Secondly, psychiatric patients suffer from illnesses which because of their nature have been poorly categorised and defined; and their outcome and characteristics are greatly influenced by personality structure and by social, educational, cultural and ageing factors. The greatest concordance is found in organic psychoses and this is followed by the functional psychoses. Poorest concordance is found in the neuroses and personality disorders. Attempts to improve reliability with use of the structured mental state interview have continued during the 1970s. The best known structured mental state interviews is the

Present State Examination (P.S.E.) which was used in the World Health Organisation pilot study of schizophrenia and in the United States — United Kingdom diagnostic project. There is an increasing emphasis on the use of a formulation rather than on diagnosis alone, as this allows greater scope for consideration of diagnostic possibilities and conveys more information on the likely course an illness will follow and the prospects for treatment. It must also be considered that while first encounter psychiatric diagnoses may be unreliable, most psychiatrists get the opportunity of gaining a fuller understanding of their patient's problem over a period of time so that the diagnosis can remain under review, and that while diagnoses may differ there is much greater conformity on management.

Q5.
Briefly the essence of Szasz's teaching is that there is no scientific foundation for ascribing the word 'disease' to most of the conditions encountered in psychiatric practice. He bases his views on the argument that there has been complete failure to demonstrate brain lesions in most of these so called 'diseases'. In relation to these views he has become an arch critic of most forms of involuntary hospitalisation, and he has had considerable influence on medico-legal thinking in the United States of America. Szasz argues further that a role behaviour model is more appropriate than a medical model for explaining psychiatric conditions. Most biologically orientated psychiatrists have responded to Szasz's views by stating that while distinct biological abnormalities cannot be found for most psychiatric conditions that does not mean that they do not exist. They express the view that psychiatric illnesses are epiphenomena of still undiscovered biological abnormalities. Such a view is consistent with the tradition of medical progress as most medical maladies were described before their etiology was clear, and on the practical level one is not justified on humanitarian grounds in allowing grossly disturbed schizophrenic or hypomanic patients unlimited freedom in a community which may be uncaring.

Q6.
Krepelin and Bleuler established the concept of schizophrenia. Krepelin's symptoms of schizophrenia (dementia praecox) included the following:- emotional blunting, lack of insight, delusions, hallucinations, negativism and stereotypies, thought disorder and lack of interest in the outside world. He also stressed the characteristic of onset in early adult life and the generally poor prognosis. Bleuler divided his criteria into primary, i.e. originating from the dis-

ease process itself and secondary criteria which were non-specific, but could be understood in the context of a reaction to the primary criteria, The primary criteria which are often called the four As are, altered affectivity, ambivalence, autism and altered associations. Secondary criteria include delusions and hallucinations. Krepelin recognised three distinct forms of schizophrenia, namely catatonic, hebephrenic and paranoid and Bleuler described a fourth — simple schizophrenia. The reliability with which patients are assigned to the various sub-categories is so low that in general the distinctions are not regarded as of much value. A more recent set of criteria has been proposed by Feighner. Very briefly, he states that it is necessary to have a chronic illness of at least six months duration at the time of evaluation and there must be an absence of depressive or manic symptoms to such an extent that an affective illness is excluded. The patient must also have one of the following — delusions or hallucinations without significant associated perplexity or disorientation, or verbal communication that makes logical understanding difficult. If three of the following manifestations are also present with the above then Feighner proposes that a diagnosis of definite schizophrenia can be made, if only two are present the diagnosis is probable — these criteria are: (a) single status (b) poor premorbid social adjustment or work history (c) family history of schizophrenia (d) absence of alcoholism or drug abuse within a year of onset (e) onset of illness prior to the age of 40.

Q7.

The impetus for doing a diagnostic project in the United States and the United Kingdom arose from the observation that the first admission rates are higher for schizophrenia in the United States than in England and that for affective disorder the first admission rates for England are higher. It was thought that this was due to differences in diagnostic evaluation rather than differences in incidences, and the project was formulated to test this hypothesis. It was found that New York city psychiatrists diagnosed schizophrenia more frequently and affective disorder less frequently than psychiatrists in London, but when standarised interviews were used (Present State Examination) the two diagnoses were found to be in much the same proportions in both cities.

Q8.

The prognosis is in all probability excellent based on the observation that she has been well for 13 years, has held down a responsible job, is well adjusted socially and now appears to be a mature personality.

Course and management

The patient was discharged and no future psychiatric involvement is envisaged.

Further reading

Copeland J 1978 Psychiatric diagnosis and classification. In: Gaind R N, Hudson B L (eds) Current themes in psychiatry, Macmillan Press Ltd, London and Basingstoke

Kendall R 1972 Schizophrenia: the remedy for dignostic confusion. Brit J Hosp Med 8: 383–390

Mullen P 1979 The phenomenology of disordered mental function. In: Hill, Murrray, Thorley (eds) Essentials of postgraduate psychiatry, Academic Press, London, New York, p 33–34

Roth M 1976 Schizophrenia and the theories of Thomas Szasz, Brit J Psychiat. 129: 317–.326

CASE 33

A 24-year-old girl with a psychiatric history and who has been diagnosed as schizophrenic is brought to outpatients by her parents. She declares that she has broken her relationship with her boy-friend with whom she has lived for two years, but says, 'I have taken up with another boy because he has a charm necklace of a stallion and he was born in the Chinese year of the snake which does not go with water, so he can treat my schizophrenia'. The father is a bus driver and the mother does part-time domestic work, there is one older sister in the family who is a state enrolled nurse. There is no history of psychiatric illness in the immediate family, but a first cousin of the patient has been treated for schizophrenia. The patient had a normal childhood, with no behavioural disorders or neurotic traits and got on well with her mother, but not so well with her father whom she describes as, 'touchy and authoritarian' and 'he ordered me out of the house on more than one occasion'. She got on well at school and left school at the age of 16, was usually about middle of the class at examinations, but did not do 'O' levels. She trained as a dressmaker for two years but did not qualify and subsequently worked in a clothes shop as a sales girl for a year, but found she didn't like it and hasn't worked outside the home since. Occasionally clothes are sent to her at home for altering, but her mother says this is now very infrequent as she has become very slow in working over the last two or three years. Up to the age of about 19 or 20 she got on well with people and was friendly and outgoing with an interest in dancing, music and boy-friends. Since the onset of her psychiatric illness at the age of 21 she has become more retiring and withdrawn although she has had two long relationships with men, the present one of about two years duration. He is a manual worker and described by the mother as very tolerant and understanding of the patient, although she is very slow and inefficient in keeping house, shopping and cooking, he has remained faithful and knows that she has a psychiatric history. There is no relevant medical history. At the age of 21 she was admitted to a psychiatric hospital for the first time, when she was described as 'depressed and slowed up' by the relatives, her appetite was poor and she had lost a stone in weight and spent long periods alone in her room. On examination she was found to have Schneiderian first rank symptoms of schizophrenia such as auditory hallucinations in the form of voices commenting on her behaviour and a feeling that she was under the control of a spirit who was able to influence her behaviour. She responded to a combination of an intra-muscular neuroleptic and oral antipsychotics and was discharged on flupenthixol 40 mg every three weeks. She remained well on this for about two and a half years, but in the two to three months preceding her outpatient's appointment she started attending a spiritualist who advised her to cease taking medication and she refused to take further injections or attend outpatients. The parents describe her as becoming 'more withdrawn and very bizarre in her speech'. Difficulties developed in her relationship with the boy-friend and she was inclined to stay in bed unduly long. She also started to smoke hashish and to stay up late at night. On admission she was found to be exhibiting Schneiderian first rank symptoms of schizophrenia — she thought she heard the voice of Jesus commenting on her behaviour, and also believed that her behaviour was controlled by a man she met with a pendant depicting a stallion. She was also insightless, had marked psychomotor retardation, there was gross blunting of affect, and she exhibited prolonged hand washing, which took up to half an hour, and she declared that this was an effort to ensure general cleanliness. She was not depressed, and her condition as far as could be ascertained, was not drug induced.

Questions

1. What is your formulation on this patient?

2. How important in this patient's relapse was her decision to cease taking a long acting neuroleptic?

3. What is the role of pharmacokinetics in monitoring treatment in psychiatry?

4. What do you mean by the term 'a superimposed obsessive compulsive symptom complex' in the context of this case?

5. In which psychiatric conditions are disturbances of mono-amine oxidase functioning postulated?

6. What do you know of the international pilot study on schizophrenia?

7. Very briefly give a critical comment on the concept of schizophrenia as purely a functional disorder.

8. Briefly criticise the hypothesis of dopaminergic overactivity in schizophrenia.

Answers

Q1.

This patient is suffering from a relapse in her schizophrenic state, with disturbances in perception, thought, affect and psychomotor activity. There is also a superimposed obsessive compulsive symptom complex, exhibited in the form of prolonged hand washing rituals. The patient's refusal to continue with medication may have been a factor in her deterioration and the acuteness of symptoms and her history of a good response to pharmacotherapy suggests that at least for the immediate future the prognosis is reasonably good, with treatment. She should be admitted to hospital and her former treatment programme should be resumed.

Q2.

It is difficult to say in the individual case how important a factor is omission of neuroleptics in the relapse of a schizophrenic patient. This patient's decision to cease taking medication and seek the help of a spiritualist may have been an indication that the patient was unwell even before she stopped medication. However, it has been observed that nearly 70 per cent of psychotic patients on placebo relapsed within nine months compared to only 8 per cent on active drugs. In a patient like this long term treatment would appear to be advisable.

Q3.

Pharmacokinetics is concerned with the study of the absorption, the metabolism, and the plasma levels in relation to particular dosages of drugs with their efficacy and their excretion. In psychiatry pharmacokinetics has so far found its most useful role in monitoring the plasma levels of lithium, and it has also been used in attempts to relate the plasma levels of tricyclic antidepressants to their efficacy. It is unlikely, however, in the foreseeable future that pharmacokinetics will play such a central role in psychiatry as it does in general medicine, where, in general, etiology and symptomatology are more precise and the effects of drugs more predictable. It must be remembered that many factors apart from the use of a specific drug at a specific dosage may determine outcome of treatment in psychiatry. Although pharmacokinetics so far (apart from lithium estimations) has not greatly influenced psychiatric clinical practice, it is useful in monitoring unexpected drug responses in individual patients.

Q4.

Obsessional and compulsive symptoms may appear in various organic brain lesions and in post encephalithic states. Also, in some patients with psychotic depression and in some with schizophrenia there appears to be a relationship between the psychosis and obsessional symptoms. Obsessional symptoms have been observed in between 3–4 per cent of hospitalised schizophrenic patients and these symptoms are observed either before or at the time of onset of the psychosis. It is possible that the obsessional rituals reflect an attempt by certain personalities to ward off or cope with the anxiety associated with the impending disorder of thought and perception found in schizophrenia. The exact relationship is, however, unknown, and there is no evidence to suggest that obsessional neurotics have a tendency to develop schizophrenia. In the context of this case the obsessive compulsive features could be regarded as a psychological reaction to the schizophrenic process.

Q5.

Disturbances in mono amine oxidase (M.A.O.) activity have been postulated in depressive illness and in schizophrenia. In affective illnesses there is some evidence to suggest that increased M.A.O. activity is present, with the result that there is a reduction in the level of biogenic amines in certain effector sites in the brain and this results in depression. There is not sufficient evidence at present to refute or support this view, and apart from the use of M.A.O.I. drugs in treatment, this line of research is not at present fruitful. In schizophrenia it has been observed that there were low levels of M.A.O. in platelets, but, in general, studies in this field are inconclusive. Reduction in M.A.O. levels were also observed in the platelets of identical schizophrenic twins even in those who did not have the illness, and low levels of M.A.O. are found more often in chronic than in acute schizophrenia. The role of M.A.O., if any, in the etiology of schizophrenia is unclear, and it may be that some abnormality of M.A.O. may be a predisposing factor to psychiatric illness in general. So far no practical benefits to schizophrenic patients have resulted from this research.

Q6.
The international pilot study of schizophrenia was carried out with the collaboration of the World Health Organisation in 1973. Nine different countries and 1202 patients were involved. The countries included three European countries, four developing countries and the United States and Russia. The primary aim was to test how the concept and the diagnostic criteria of schizophrenia varied internationally. The results showed that the European and the developing countries had similar diagnostic criteria for schizophrenia but the criteria were much broader in the United States and Russia.

Q7.
The concept of schizophrenia as purely a functional disorder has survived mainly because no consistent demonstrable neuropathology has been disclosed and at least up to recently, no demonstrable consistent biochemical abnormality of the nervous system could be incriminated with any degree of certainty, as being of etiological importance. Scrutiny of the literature, however, discloses that there are reports of dilated ventricles in schizophrenic brains, e.g. in a minority of institutionalised schizophrenics with cognitive impairment, dilated ventricles were demonstrated on C.A.T. scans. It must also be remembered that the association of schizophrenia with many organic nervous system disorders exceeds chance expectations and that the association of schizophrenic-like psychoses with temporal lobe epilepsy has been reasonably well established and up to 80 per cent of psychotic epileptics have an abnormal temporal lobe focus. Although advances in biochemical investigations of the C.N.S. may disclose more subtle abnormalities in schizophrenia, it would be naive to embrace a purely organic or functional concept, as there will always be an onus on the individual to interact and function at some level with society, so that the organic and functional aspects of the condition will always have to be considered.

Q8.
The hypothesis of dopaminergic overactivity in schizophrenia can be criticised on the observation that estimates of dopamine turnover by the measurement of dopamine metabolites in both schizophrenic brains at autopsy and in C.S.F. from schizophrenic patients does not provide direct evidence for central dopaminergic overactivity. The possibility that relative dopaminergic overactivity occurs with deficiences in antagonistic neurotransmitter systems or with abnormalities in substances which influence the effects of dopamine has

not been excluded. It is unknown why there is a delay in producing clinical improvement in schizophrenic patients by administering neuroleptics, when it is known from animal studies that neuroleptics have an acute action in producing dopamine receptor blockade. It is quite possible that a primary antipsychotic effect is not due to dopamine blockade but to adaptive biochemical changes, which occur over the latent period in response to dopamine blockade. It is speculative what the exact functioning relationship of dopamine is with such substances as the morphine-like peptide beta-endorphin or noradrenaline in the etiology of schizophrenia. It has been suggested that a deficiency of endogenous brain peptides similar to beta-endorphin is associated with schizophrenia. It has also been suggested that dopamine and noradrenaline, both neurotransmitters, may act synergistically. It is quite possible that schizophrenia is a non-specific entity and includes a variety of conditions with heterogenous biochemical abnormalities of which absolute or relative dopaminergic overactivity is but one feature of some.

Course and management

The patient was admitted to hospital and a long acting I.M. neuroleptic flupenthixol 40 mg once two weekly was prescribed and the patient improved considerably. After five weeks she was discharged and continued with treatment and attended outpatients.

Further reading

Campbell I C 1981 Blood platelets and psychiatry. Brit J Psychiat 138: 78–80

Cheung H K 1981 Schizophrenics fully remitted on neuroleptics for three to five years, to stop or continue drugs. Brit J Psychiat 138: 490–495

Rosen I 1957 The clinical significance of obsessions in schizophrenia. J Ment Sci 103: 773–786

Spokes E G S 1978 Current biochemical theories of schizophrenia. In: Edwards G (ed) Current themes in schizophrenia, University of Southampton, Southampton, p 6–26

CASE 34

A 62-year-old man is referred to outpatients of a psychiatric hospital from a general hospital, presents in a confused restless manner and is verbally aggressive when prevented from wandering. There is no coherent history available from the patient, and his medical history says that four months previously he was involved in a road traffic accident and sustained severe head injuries, with fracture of the left tempero-frontal area of the skull with considerable contusion of the left tempero-frontal area of the brain and bleeding into the C.S.F. This resulted in a variable and fluctuating level of consciousness for two days. He regained full consciousness after the depressed segment of bone was elevated and he now has a right hemiparesis and is markedly dysphasic. His daughter says he was well up to the time of the accident and he has no previous psychiatric history. He worked as a carpenter all his life, retired two years previously and has worked part time since then. There are two other children in the family and his marriage is described as successful. He was interested in sport and television, smoked and drank moderately and is described as a 'warm outgoing personality'. He has enjoyed robust physical health. On assessment he is restless and agitated and appears to be confused. He can follow commands but exhibits marked dysphasia, it is possible however, to interpret his replies to questions. He attempts to leave the clinical room repeatedly and has to be continually requested to return. His cognitive functioning is difficult to assess, but he is probably confused. He failed to learn the layout of his previous ward on which he spent two months, and was inclined to wander off and get lost. There is no evidence of affective or perceptual disturbance. Physical examination confirms a right hemiparesis, he is resistive to examination, is inclined to react aggressively and attempts to suck the patella hammer.

Questions

1. What is your formulation on this patient?

2. What are the immediate psychiatric sequelae of severe head injury?

3. What are the remote psychiatric sequelae of severe head injury?

4. Would you distinguish between post traumatic neurosis and the post traumatic syndrome?

5. Is there a relationship between the socio-psychiatric background of parents and the risk of accidents to children?

6. What is the underlying cerebral pathology and the psychiatric features of the punch drunk syndrome (chronic traumatic encephalopathy of boxers)?

7. How would you assess the psychiatric prognosis for this patient?

Answers

Q1.

This 62-year-old patient suffered severe brain injury due to a road traffic accident, resulting in motor, intellectual and personality impairment. At present he is in need of psychiatric supervision in a hospital setting and it is likely he will need ongoing care. It is possible though unlikely at this stage that he will show such spontaneous improvement in his intellectual functioning and behavioural pattern that treatment in the community could be considered. Nevertheless gradual improvements can be observed even over a period of years. While in hospital it would be advisable for him to have psychometric testing at regular intervals to monitor his intellectual functioning, physiotherapy to maximise his movements, and a trial of various psychotropic drugs to see which is most appropriate to control his restlessness and occasional aggressive behaviour.

Q2.

The immediate psychiatric consequence of severe head injury is dominated by varying levels of impaired consciousness. Throughout this period there is impaired registration of events with the result that there is marked post traumatic amnesia and confusion and the duration of this amnesia is often directly related to the severity of the brain damage. Agitation, restlessness and aggressive and violent behaviour may be observed. If the patient can complain he may comment on a feeling of restlessness and giddiness, of irritability, forgetfulness and apprehension in the face of unaccustomed tasks. There may be pervasive overriding anxiety about the injury and marked emotional responses to it. Emotional lability may be present.

Q3.

The remote psychiatric sequelae of severe head injury include personality and intellectual deterioration, neurotic and psychotic reactions as well as the psychiatric accompaniments of traumatic epilepsy. Personality deterioration may show itself in argumentative attitudes or in aggressive and violent behaviour, and a clean efficient person may become slovenly, inefficient and neglect his personal hygiene. Left hemisphere lesions especially those involving the temporal and frontal lobes most commonly present with personality change. The degree of intellectual deterioration is very closely related to the severity of the head injury and the duration of post traumatic amnesia. Post traumatic amnesia greater than 24 hours duration suggests that the long term intellectual prognosis is poor. There may be marked disturbance in recent and remote memory, new material is not registered and recalled, and confusion will be marked. The term post traumatic neuroses can encompass the complete range of neurotic disorders, including depressive, hysterical and obsessional reactions and anxiety states. There is frequently prominent agitation, restlessness and hypochondriasis, with numerous somatic complaints such as headaches and dizziness. Patients seem to lack motivation and drive and complain of anergia, and emotional incontinence may be observed. It has been observed that psychotic conditions, especially schizophreniform states, develop more commonly than expected in the late post traumatic period. It is probable that the stress of the accident precipitates the psychosis in those individuals constitutionally predisposed, and damage to the temporal lobe may be an important etiological factor. Post traumatic epilepsy should it occur may be accompanied by the much discussed psychiatric complications such as psychoses, personality and behaviour problems, and the patient will have to cope with the social and occupational difficulties the epileptic faces. Epilepsy is observed in 30 per cent of severe open head injuries within a five year period.

Q4.

It may be very difficult in the individual case to distinguish between post traumatic neurosis and the post traumatic syndrome as there is considerable overlap and one may merge into the other. Post traumatic neurosis covers a wide range of neurotic conditions including obsessional and depressive states, anxiety states and hysterical reactions. The post traumatic syndrome differs in that

   a. It is more circumscribed and characterised frequently by complaints of imparied concentration, restlessness, intolerance of noise and generally a very low frustration level.

b. It is to be observed in more minor degrees of head injury.
c. It may be associated with premorbid vulnerable personality types who would be positively re-inforced by injury to adopt the sick role in order to gain financial rewards.

Q5.
It has been observed that working class children are more at risk from accidents than middle class children and psychiatric disorder in the parents has also been linked to increased risk. From the social aspects the risk appears to be related to such factors as overcrowding, large families and unemployment of the father. Psychiatric illness in the mother especially depression also greatly increases the risk of accidents to children. Psychiatric disorder in the mother is thought to provoke a change in behaviour in the child characterised by extroversion, aggression, impulsiveness and daring and this exposes the child to hazards. There is no evidence to support the view that by exposing himself to increased danger from accidents, the child deliberately attempts to provoke or punish the parent.

Q6.
The punch drunk syndrome (chronic traumatic encephalopathy of boxers) becomes noticeable, with neurological and psychiatric features prominent, towards the end of some boxers' careers. The condition results from brain damage by rotational-accleration forces sustained at the moment of successive blows to the head. Pathologically in well developed cases there is diffuse neuronal loss especially in the medial temporal cortex and the hippocampus. The floor of the hypothalamus is thinned, the fornices are torn from their attachments and the mammilliary bodies are sunken. Psychiatrically paranoid delusions of financial exploitation or marital infidelity may be prominent, there may be intellectual impairment, poor memory and recall. Personality deterioration may also be observed and this is characterised by explosive aggressive behaviour and rage reactions. There may be poor tolerance for alcohol, which may accentuate the innate aggressive tendencies. Neurological signs of pyramidal, extra pyramidal, and cerebellar origin may ante-date the psychiatric features.

Q7.
There are some guidelines for assessing the prognosis for psychiatric disorder associated with head injuries. In general the more severe the injury, and the longer the period of post traumatic amnesia, the worse the prognosis. Open head injuries tend to have a poorer prog-

nosis, than closed ones, as the likelihood of traumatic epilepsy is increased. Younger patients in general do better. Patients of poor premorbid personality do not recover as well or as quickly as good premorbid personalities. Although improvement in psychiatric conditions associated with head injuries can occur for over a year or more after the injury, if there is no improvement within the first six months this is of poor prognostic significance. Severe neurological deficit is directly related to severity of brain injury and indicates poor prognosis for accompanying psychiatric states. The prognosis for this patient would therefore be poor on the basis of the severity of his head injury, his age and the absence of any detectable improvement over a four month period. It is likely that ongoing hospital care will be indicated.

Course and management

The patient was admitted to hospital for assessment and observation and if necessary to formulate a long term care programme. He needed ongoing care.

Further reading

Brown G W, Davidson S 1978 Social class psychiatric disorder of parents and accidents to children. Lancet 1: 378–381

Connolly J 1981 Accident proneness. Brit J Hosp Med 26(5): 470–481

Corrsellis J A N, Bristow C J, Freeman-Brown D 1973 The aftermath of boxing. Psych Med 3: 270–303

Lishman W A 1973 The psychiatric sequelae of head injury. Psych Med 3: 304–318

Milller H 1961 Accident neurosis. Brit Med J 1: 919–925, 992, 998

CASE 35

A 22-year-old girl is referred to a psychiatric hospital from a general hospital, where she had been admitted three days previously after she had an 'epileptiform attack'. Her 'fit' was thought to be related to alcohol withdrawal and she was referred to the psychiatric hospital because she was considered to be in need of help with an alcohol problem. Her parents are alive, the father is a retired clerk, she lives with them and has one older brother who is married. There is no history of psychiatric illness in the family but the mother was recently treated with diazepam by her general practitioner because of 'nervous tension' caused by the patient's behaviour. The patient had a normal childhood, there were no neurotic traits and she attended school from five until the age of 17, was reasonably bright and did two 'O' levels one in English and one in Geography. She had the menarche at 11 and her periods are regular but painful and she received sex education from her school mates and her parents, she is heterosexual and met her first boyfriend when she was 17. According to herself she is, 'a warm friendly personality and I make friends easily'. She was never involved with the police. Her physical health is good, but she had a previous psychiatric admission to hospital for the treatment of anorexia nervosa when she was 19. When some of her friends started to diet she joined them and her weight went from 10 stone down to six and a half stone and she experienced amenorrhoea and if pressurized to eat she would later induce vomiting. She responded to hospitalization, bed rest, supervised eating and tranquillisers and reached nine and a half stone, since then her weight has remained stable. After leaving school she trained as a clerk/receptionist and held down a senior secretarial post in a hotel for two years. While in this post she started to drink excessively and was finally sacked for absenteeism. She next worked in a bar and her heavy drinking continued. Her drinking pattern is characterised by long periods of abstinence which are followed by binges of a few days, when she would drink up to a bottle of spirits a day plus some lager. These drinking bouts may occur up to three times monthly. Eventually she lost her job in the pub because of her drinking behaviour and for the last seven months has not worked. During this period there has been considerable friction at home between her and her parents who strongly disapprove of her drinking behaviour. On the day prior to admission to the general hospital she had no alcohol intake after a heavy drinking bout from the previous two days, she felt 'tense, nervous and jittery' and eventually had 'a fit'. On assessment she appears well physically, is not depressed or suicidal, and appears to be of good intellectual level. Psychometric testing shows her to be in the high average range with no organic impairment but with evidence of depression.

Questions

1. What is your formulation on this patient?

2. Which psychological tests might a psychologist use in assessing this patient's intellectual level, her affective state, her personality and the presence or absence of organic cerebral deterioration?

3. Very briefly what do you know of the familial, occupational and sexual complications of alcoholism?

4. What is your concept of anorexia nervosa?

5. Is there evidence for primary hypothalamic malfunction in anorexia nervosa?

6. What effect may psychiatric illness in a member have on the family?

7. Very briefly comment from a psychiatric viewpoint on the statement, 'It is a pity that youth is wasted on the young'.

8. How would you treat this patient?

Answers

Q1.

This patient is suffering from a severe alcohol related problem, characterised by frequent bouts of heavy prolonged drinking followed by periods of abstinence. As a result of this behaviour she has lost her occupation on two occasions and her familial relationship with her parents has deteriorated. There is no obvious underlying psychiatric disorder on clinical evaluation, but psychometric testing suggests that she may be depressed, and there is a history of psychiatric hospitalisation for the treatment of anorexia nervosa. The prognosis will depend to a large extent on the adequacy of the patient's personality and her willingness to co-operate with treatment. Ameliorating prognostic factors include the patient's youth, the absence of alcohol related physical and mental damage and the ongoing contact with her family.

Q2.

There are a variety of tests available to the psychologist. Intellectual deterioration can be measured by the Babcock test and the Shipley-Hartford test. In assessing intellectual level the Wais Adult Intelligence Scale (W.A.I.S.) is probably the most commonly used test. In testing for depression the Hamilton Rating Scale (H.R.S.), the Beck Depression Inventory (B.D.I.), the Zung Self-Rating Depression Scale or the British Hospital Progress Test could be used. Personality assessment tests commonly used are the Eysenck Personality Inventory (E.P.I.) or the Minnesota Multiphasic Personality Inventory (M.M.P.I.) and projective tests which include the Rorschach and the Thematic Apperception Tests. Test of organic deterioration include the Wechsler Deterioration Indices, and verbal learning tests such as the modified word learning test and the paired associate learning test. The experienced psychologist will use the most appropriate battery of tests for each individual and will be able to inter-relate the results and in conjunction with relevant clinical information give a helpful report.

Q3.

Alcoholism gives rise to serious familial, occupational and social problems. It is an important cause of marital breakdown, divorce and wife battering, and may have an adverse influence on the developing personalities of children. There is very substantial evidence that in alcohol dependent pregnant women the foetus is at special risk from cardiovascular defects, retarded growth and development (foetal alcohol syndrome). Alcoholics also have two to three times as many days off work as their non-dependent colleagues, they are also much more likely to have been sacked on one or more occasions, and are less likely to achieve promotion or progress in their careers. Sexually there is a falling off of interest, and although alcohol may stimulate sexual desire, the ability to perform the act is diminished, and this may lead to frustration, anger and violence in the intoxicated individual. Many patients exhibiting morbid jealousy are also either alcoholic or gross abusers of alcohol, and controlled subconscious sexual problems such as latent homosexuality may become overt.

Q4.

Classically, anorexia nervosa is a disorder of adolescent or young women, characterised by severe dieting, with gross weight loss, amenorrhoea and an accompanying increase rather than decrease in physical activity. The patient will go to great lengths to avoid food intake and will induce vomiting or secrete food away if not observed. The etiology of the condition is unknown. It has been suggested that it represents an assertion of independence by the young person, a rejection of parental control, and by influencing the form of her body, she exhibits a type of power and control. It has also been suggested that anorexics have a false perception of their body image and perceive themselves as fatter than normal. It is also thought that anorexia nervosa may be a symptom of an underlying phobia of normal female adolescent weight gain associated with pubertal changes. The possibility that there is a physical cause for the condition has not been excluded and most attention has centred on hypothalamic functioning. More recently considerable interest has focussed on the family dynamics of these patients.

Q5.

Interest on hypothalamic function in anorexia nervosa has arisen because it is the centre for the control of appetite and endocrine regulation. The problem is whether any observed disorder of hypothalamic function is primary or secondary to the anorexic state. Weight gain results in the correction of most associated psychological abnormalities but an abnormality in the cyclical fluctuating concentrations of gonadotrophins persists. Also the expected release of luteinising hormone after a course of oestrogens is not observed. These observations suggest that there is a primary disorder of hypothalamic functioning, but it does not exclude the possibility that the hypothalamus may have suffered irreparable damage during dieting, or that attainment of normal weight may still be accompanied by irregular eating patterns and emotional upset.

Q6.

Psychiatric illness in a family member may place considerable strain on the family unit and in some cases threatens its existence. The effects will be determined by the type, severity and duration of the illness, the strengths, weaknessess and tolerance threshold of the family and the extent of community and hospital supportive facilities available. Alcohol and other drug dependent states are particularly destructive of family cohesion and when occurring in a marriage partner may lead to violence, separation and divorce. Patients categorised as psychopathic, many of whom also abuse drugs or alcohol, may be profoundly disruptive of family equilibrium. Psychotic illnesses and schizophrenia in particular may place ongoing stress on the family, and this is rather marked when the patient lives within the jurisdiction of a psychiatric service which emphasises extra-mural care. There will be loss of social and leisure activities, occupational activities of family members may be upset, with loss of earnings. Many families of schizophrenic patents carry great burdens uncomplainingly. Patients suffering from dementias of various kinds place considerable burdens on families. The degrading aspects of the illness is distressful to relatives, the wandering, the dangerous and unpredictable use of gas and electricity, the various forms of incontinence, emotional, faecal and urinary, causes worry and upset. Admission to hospital of an elderly demented parent may be associated with considerable guilt and grief in the relatives.

Q7.
This statement could be regarded as fair comment by a middle aged psychiatrist in a cynical mood. Accidents, psychopathic behaviour, drug and alcohol abuse, violent and irresponsible social and sexual behaviour, and crime are common among the young. These behaviour patterns occur when the individuals are enjoying robust physical health and are at their optimum cerebral and intellectual functioning level and are most idealistic and so would be well endowed to engage in worthwhile social, humanitarian or artistic endeavour. To espouse this view wholeheartedly, however, would not only be cynical, but simplistic psychiatrically. Only a minority of young people engage in these activities. The young individual is not only a product of his genetic endowment, but also of the influences of school, family and peers during his developmental period, so to a large degree his behaviour patterns are determined by adults. Youth, like other periods of life is a learning period, a time of trial and error, and most young people pass through it wiser and undamaged. The inference in the statement is that the endowments of youth would be much better used by the middle aged or the old. These age groups may be characterised by rigidity, inflexibility, lack of originality and idealism and to invest them with robust physical and intellectual power might be a dubious investment.

Q8.
This patient should be admitted for further assessment and the extent of her alcohol related problem should be investigated. Management

and prognosis will depend to a large extent on her insight and willingness to accept help and change her life style. Should she be willing to accept help then there are a variety of inpatient and outpatient support facilities available. Within the hospital any associated psychiatric problem such as depression should be treated, group therapy referral may be indicated and career guidance and retraining for an occupation after discharge may also be indicated. Aversion therapy and/or one of the anti-alcohol drugs such as disulfiram (Antabuse) may reinforce the patient's good intentions. On discharge from hospital, attendance at psychiatric outpatients would be advisable and referral to Alcoholics Anonymous may be appropriate.

Course and management

This patient discharged herself against medical advice after eight days in hospital, and refused to consider outpatient management.

Further reading

Beaumont P J V 1979 The endocrinology of anorexia nervosa. In: Granville Grossman K (ed) Recent advances in clinical psychiatry 3, Churchill Livingstone, Edinburgh, London, New York, p 210–216

Dally P 1981 Treatment of anorexia nervosa. Brit J Hosp Med 25(5): 434–443

Pai S, Kapur R L 1981 The burden on the family of a psychiatric patient: development of an interview schedule. Brit J Psychiat 138: 332–335

Russell G F M 1977 Editorial-The present state of anorexia nervosa. Psych Med 7: 363–367

CASE 36

A 56-year-old married woman is referred by her general practitioner with a two-year history of repeated checking to ensure that, for example, windows are shut, gas and water taps turned off. She has a fear of harm coming to her son, daughter-in-law and grandchildren and attributes most of her checking to this e.g. in case she inadvertently leaves a gas tap turned on and they are affected. She realises that her fears and her behaviour are irrational and tries to ignore the former but becomes increasingly anxious if she does not check, and irritated if she is interrupted in the process. The patient's parents died within four weeks of each other about three years ago and her husband feels that she has changed since then, becoming upset easily and losing interest in things. 14 years ago her 12-year-old daughter died from a staphylococcal enteritis following appendicitis and the patient tended to blame herself for the death and has continued to do so despite reassurance from her husband. He believes she has never really accepted the loss and, for example, has kept the daughter's clothes and for a long time refused to have a grave stone placed on the grave. There is no known family history of psychiatric illness and she describes a happy childhood with good relationships with her parents and siblings. After leaving school at the age of 14 where she was rather backward and largely unable to write, she worked chiefly as a shop assistant until recently when her work in a mail order firm has involved checking application forms and letters at which she tends to be slow. Her periods started at the age of 13 and ceased nine years ago. She married at the age of 19 to a coach builder whom she had known for four years. The marriage is a happy one but she has been less interested in the sexual relationship since the death of the daughter. The son is now aged 31 and is married with two children. There is no past medical or psychiatric history of significance. In her personality she describes herself as shy, introverted and a perfectionist. She is very conscientious with the housework but does not like her flat because it is in a district associated with a lot of theft, and mugging, and she and her husband have been trying to move for two years to be nearer to the son. Enlarging on her problem, she describes a daily routine before going to work, lasting an hour, in which she checks the whole house — going from room to room, spending about 10 minutes at a window trying to convince herself that it is properly shut. All this is, however, much reduced at weekends when her husband is present and able to reassure her. She describes feelings of depression at times but her sleep and appetite are unimpaired. On examination she appears a slightly depressed lady of probably below average intelligence but with no other abnormality in the mental state.

Questions

1. What is the diagnosis or differential diagnosis in this patient?

2. What likely etiological factors would you consider with this patient?

3. In which psychiatric conditions may you find obsessive compulsive symptoms?

4. What is the classic psychoanalytical view of obsessional neurosis?

5. How would you manage this patient?

6. Is severe neurosis associated with premature mortality?

7. Comment briefly on the statement, 'This woman's anxiety will invariably be relieved by obsessive compulsive rituals'.

8. What precisely is meant by 'categories of obsessional patients'?

9. Is resistance invariably found in obsessional illness?

Answers

Q1.

The clinical picture is dominated by the patient's obsessive-compulsive checking rituals. These are secondary to the primary obsessional fear that harm may come to others. This is obsessional since:

   a. The recurrent thoughts or fears intrude into her awareness against her wishes and she tries to resist them.

   b. She realises their irrationality.

   c. She becomes increasingly anxious until she is able to calm her fears by the secondary compulsive checking.

These features distinguish the obsessional phenomena from:

   a. Phobic anxiety in which the patient fears some harm may befall him in particular situations.

b. A preoccupation, for example with thoughts of past misdeeds, in a patient with a depressive illness.

c. Thought insertion in schizophrenia when the patient believes thoughts are being inserted into his mind by some outside agency.

In this patient the differential diagnosis lies between an obsessional per se or a depressive illness with marked obsessional features though there is no evidence of the physiological accompaniments (sleep and appetite disturbance etc.) of a depressive illness.

Q2.

There is no evidence here of any genetic contribution but the nature of the illness is certainly consistent with the patient's previous rather obsessional personality. From the history, and especially from the husband's account, it seems likely that this patient has an unresolved grief reaction to the death of her daughter 14 years previously and that this has been exacerbated by the more recent loss of both parents. She still blames herself for the death and, psychodynamically it may be supposed that she unconsciously believes that she could be responsible for further deaths and so has to counteract this by obsessional checking. Additional stresses may include the environmental difficulties associated with the flat and the obsessional nature of the patient's present work.

Q3.

Obsessive compulsive symptoms may be found in the course of almost any mental illness. They are most commonly associated with anxiety and depressive states. Quite frequently they are seen in the setting of schizophrenia and also in brain damaged patients.

Q4.

In the classic psychoanalytic view a spectrum ranging from obsessional traits to obsessional personality and on to obsessional disorder is described. It is postulated that all these states reflect a regression to anal sadism. Obsessive compulsive disorder does not always arise within an obsessive personality type, just as a conversion reaction does not always arise within a hysterical personality. The individual tries to control his environment by his rituals, just as the child at the anal stage of development tries to control his environment and people in it by opening or refusing to open his bowels. Unacceptable ideas for the super ego arising from id are the repressed and replaced by acceptable ideas or rituals, and the ego is protected, but unconscious conflict remains unresolved.

Q5.

The more that the obsessional picture is based on a depressive illness the better since the latter may respond fairly rapidly to antidepressant treatment. For this reason, since this patient certainly describes a depressed mood, it might be worth prescribing an antidepressant drug as a therapeutic trial. At the same time she will need help to deal with the unresolved grief reaction and should be encouraged to talk of the loss and her feelings about it with the aim of reaching a more realistic appraisal of its meaning and her own relationship to it. To deal with the obsessional rituals a behavioural approach might be attempted with the object of achieving an association between a feeling of relaxation and those situations previously evoking checking behaviour, though limited intelligence and insight could make this difficult. Finally, help might be given in the way of a letter to the Housing association supporting a transfer to accommodation nearer to her son and his family.

Q6.

There is considerable evidence suggesting that severe neurosis is associated with marked premature mortality. This appears to be particularly valid for hospitalised neurotics. Although a large part of this mortality is due to accidents and suicide there is still a major excess of deaths from nervous, circulatory and respiratory diseases. It is unclear to what degree the increased mortality can be explained by the diagnosis of neurosis at the time of undiagnosed concurrent serious physical illnesses, or whether neurosis predisposes to the development of a serious illness or renders the prognosis less favourable due to non-compliance with treatment.

Q7.

Obsessive compulsive rituals are certainly of great importance in relieving anxiety and they serve that function in this patient. It has been observed, however, that rituals are not always anxiolytic, and it has been noted that some 'hand washers' feel more anxious not less during their ritual. If an individual is interrupted during the ritual, as in the case of the present patient, great irritation and anxiety may be generated. It is not uncommon to find patients burdened with external stress and increasing anxiety related to family, jobs, or examinations, ritualising less not more. The relationship of rituals to anxiety also has implications for treatment. Observations that reducing rituals led to less and not more anxiety became the basis of response prevention treatment techniques during which a patient is prevented from washing after exposure to a contaminating stimulus. The relationship is, however, complex, and some postulate a wilful aspect to the disorder, with some categories of obsessional patients seeking out contamination in order to provoke anxiety, with the symptoms viewed as a penance for bad behaviour.

Q8.

The literature contains references to sub categories of obsessional illnesses. Obsessionals have been discussed as distinct from compulsives but in general compulsive rituals are recognised as secondary to obsessional ruminations. Patients with bizarre obsessions or rituals have been described as distinct from those with more commonplace ones, such as hand-washing or gas tap checking. Acute and chronic obsessionals have been described, with the former related to environmental stress and the latter to puberty, when re-emergent sexuality is dealt with by a regression to anal sadism. It is claimed by its authors that the Maudsley Obsessional Inventory, on the basis of symptom clustering, separates obsessionals into four groups namely cleaners, checkers, ruminators and patients described as suffering from primary obsessional slowness. For example, cleaners are distinguished from checkers not only by their specific compulsion, but also in that they are more likely to be female, have a sudden onset of their symptoms and are better able to make decisions. Checking rituals are reported as less successful than cleaning varieties in relieving anxiety. Obsessional illness is probably not a homogeneous syndrome.

Q9.

Compulsion and resistance have been regarded for a long time as the two essential components of obsessive compulsive illnesses, with the recognition that the obsessions were senseless and of subsidiary importance. More recent studies have questioned the importance of resistance as many patients are described as having little or no resistance to carrying out their rituals. Some workers now think it appropriate that there should be a redefinition of obsessive compulsive neurosis with less emphasis on resistance and more on the recognition of senselessness. More precise descriptions of sub categories of obsessional illnesses will contribute substantially to clarification of the problem.

Course and management

After some explanation of the nature of staphylococcal enteritis and the fact that she could in no way have been responsible for the daughter's death she seemed reassured. Checking behaviour continued, however, and as the husband described more 'fits of depression' she was given an anti-depressant, dothiepin 25 mg t.d.s. as well as diazepam 5 mg t.d.s. With no obvious improvement two weeks later it was arranged that she should attend the day hospital. There she was assessed for behavioural treatment but the psychologist found that she was insufficiently motivated for this purpose. After two weeks in the day hospital she was keen to return to work but of a less exacting nature and this was arranged. She was followed up as an outpatient and after some weeks stopped the medication because of side effects (dry mouth). Some checking behaviour continued but to a lesser extent and she was discharged about eight months after her first attendance saying that although she was still liable to check it no longer worried her and she felt generally better in herself. She was still hoping to move.

Further reading

Insel T R 1982 Obsessive compulsive disorder — five clinical questions and a suggested approach. Comp Psychiat 23 (3): 241–251

Sims A, Prior P 1978 The pattern of mortality in severe neuroses. Brit J Psychiat 133: 299–305

Stern R S, Cobb J P 1978 The phenomenology of obsessive-compulsive neurosis. Brit J Psychiat 132: 233–239

CASE 37

A 52 year-old woman is referred by her social worker to outpatients, because she has become increasingly confused and physically incapacitated and her 21 years old bachelor son can no longer care for her. There is no family psychiatric history and neither her parents nor her sister suffered with her illness, from the patient's and the son's account. She had a happy childhood, was a good student, left school at 16, had various jobs and married at 25. She separated from her husband after 17 years of marriage. She worked as a copy typist up to seven years ago when she had to stop due to her illness. She describes her pre-morbid personality as normal and apparently there were no gross adverse personality traits. There is no previous psychiatric history but she was admitted to a general hospital five years previously with her presenting complaint. She first noticed her illness about seven years ago when there was an insidious onset of jerky unco-ordinated movements and difficulty in walking. Her symptoms progressed gradually, she began to fall and injure herself. She was also incontinent of urine partly because she could not get to the lavatory in time. She had difficulty in dressing and spilled fluids when she fed herself. The son continued to care for her at home but became increasingly anxious that she would injure herself while he was at work. At interview she is pleasant, co-operative and exhibits constant marked choreiform movements of arms and trunk and grimacing facial movements. Her speech is slurred and difficult to understand but meaningful conversation is still possible. She looks sad but denies feeling depressed. There is some cognitive impairment — she is not able to give the date, but after a delay can recall the day, month and year and can name prominent people in public life. She has difficulty in learning new material and cannot concentrate on the simplest arithmetical problems. No other abnormality is noted. Psychological assessment concluded that there was a global impairment of cognitive functioning consistent with a diagnosis of generalised organic brain disease.

Questions

1. What is the diagnosis?

2. What is the genetic basis of Huntington's chorea?

3. Are there any behavioural consequences to the illness?

4. What do you know of Huntington's chorea in the young?

5. What are the brain changes in Huntington's chorea?

6. How does the condition differ clinically and pathologically from Alzheimer's disease?

7. What is the role of genetic counselling in the prevention of Huntington's chorea?

8. How would you manage this case?

Answers

Q1.
It is most likely that this patient is suffering from Huntington's chorea, and has a typical mental and physical presentation.

Q2.
Huntington's chorea is in all probability transmitted from generation to generation by an as yet unidentified single autosomal dominant gene. This means that there is a 50 percent chance of the child of a 'carrier'parent being him or herself a bearer of the defective gene. The condition is always expressed in those with the aberrant gene.

Q3.
Apart from dementia Huntington's chorea has been associated with many types of mental distress and/or disorders. In the early stages the psychiatric sequelae of the disease may range from schizophreniform syndromes to personality changes, with behaviour disorders. Cases of irrational jealousy, paranoia and sexual disinhibition have also been reported, and suicide rates in choreic families in America are seven times the national average.

Q4.
In individuals under 30 the illness may be divided into two sub-types, clinically distinct, called juvenile Huntington's chorea and the Westphal variant. In the juvenile type, choreiform movements are rare or absent, while rigidity and epilepsy are common and dementia is more marked. Death occurs after about seven years from onset. In the Westphal type tremor is an early symptom, and muscle rig-

idity is prominent. A striking abnormality is the inability to move the eyes, thus giving the sufferer a fixed 'doll's eye' gaze.

Q5.
There is considerable brain atrophy found on post mortem, the areas most affected being the basal ganglia (which may be reduced in weight by as much as 50 percent at the time of death), the cerebellum and the brain stem adjacent to the substantia nigra. Nerve cell loss is particularly evident in the juvenile form.

Q6.
In Alzheimer's disease memory disturbance is characteristically the earliest feature of the disease, and dysphasic, apraxic, and agnosic difficulties may also be evident. Gross choreiform movements are absent in Alzheimer's Disease but in the terminal phases gross neurological disability may include spastic hemiparesis and severe striatal rigidity and tremor. In Alzheimer's disease there is gross generalised atrophy affecting most severely the frontal and temporal lobes and the most striking characteristic is the presence of senile plaques and neurofibrillary tangles.

Q7.
Each National Health Service region has its own genetic advisory service. At present the only effective means of preventing the condition is for 'at risk' individuals to remain childless. It may be necessary to tell a couple that one partner has a one in two, to one in four chance of having the choreic gene. This still leaves prospective parents with a difficult choice. There is at present no satisfactory screening test to identify those carrying the abnormal gene from their normal siblings. There is a need for educating members of choreic families, as many are ignorant of the genetic implications of their condition.

Q8.
The son is no longer able to cope with her so admission to hospital for physical and psychological assessment initially for a specified period is necessary. This would also give the son some relief. It is likely that she will soon need ongoing care in hospital or some other institution. There are no drugs which markedly influence the condition or the movements. Tetrabenazine may be worth trying to control the choreiform movements. The aim of treatment is to optimise her mental and physical capabilities and provide as congenial a life style as possible while giving relief to caring relatives.

With increasing mental and physical dependency the need for permanent hospitalisation will eventually be unavoidable.

Management and course

The patient was originally admitted for a month and was psychologically and physically assessed. She attended a rehabilitation assessment centre but was found to be too incapacitated to engage in anything but diversionary occupational therapy. She moves with the aid of a walking frame, leaves the ward to attend therapy daily and the son takes her out for weekends and holidays.

Further reading

McLellan D L, Chalmers R J, Johnson R H 1974 A double blind trial of tetrabenazine, thiopropazate and placebo in patients with chorea. Lancet 1: 104–107

Office of health economics publication 1980 Huntington's chorea. Office of health economics, 162 Regent Street, London Wir 6DD

Spokes E G S 1978 Understanding Huntington's chorea, Smith, Kline, French publications

CASE 38

A 31-year-old woman is admitted to hospital under Section 25 of the Mental Health Act at the request of her social worker because she is behaving in a psychotic manner, is deluded and hallucinated and her 29 month old daughter who lives with her is considered to be in danger. The parents are alive and well and there is no history of psychiatric illness. There is one sister who died from cirrhosis of the liver due to alcoholism and two brother who are well. She had an uncomplicated birth, had a lonely childhood, but was terrified by her parents' quarrels. She was always in the top four at school and did 'O' levels. She married at the age of 20 but divorced after two years. She cohabited with the second husband for three years before getting married five years ago, separated from him two years ago and now lives in a council flat with her daughter. When the patient was admitted to hospital, the daughter was put in foster care. The daughter had a bruise over her right eye which the patient admits to inflicting and she is not being adequately fed and clothed. Premorbidly she describes herself as a bright intelligent girl without gross neurotic traits or behaviour disorders. She smoked hashish a few times and used L.S.D. once but not within a year of admission She experienced what she described as a 'bad trip' from L.S.D. She expresses doubts about her sexual identity and admits to having difficulties in establishing an enduring relationship with men. She had four psychiatric admissions before the present one and had been diagnosed as suffering with schizophrenia and described as having a vulnerable immature personality. During one admission she was diagnosed as suffering with depression in the setting of an immature personality and responded well to antidepressants and supportive psychotherapy. At interview the patient appears lost in thought, sometimes rather depressed but becomes alert quite readily. She uses psychiatric terminology, and draws unintelligible graphs and designs to explain her thoughts and feelings. She shows objective and subjective evidence of auditory hallucinations and admits to hearing voices talking about her and believes that others can readily read her thoughts. She does not admit to feeling depressed, but her mood overall appears indifferent and flat. At times she appears to smile inappropriately and does not appear concerned about her daughter's welfare. On previous psychological testing her I.Q. was described as in the superior range.

Questions

1. What is the most likely diagnosis in this case?

2. Are you surprised that this patient appeared to respond to anti-depressant treatment on a previous admission?

3. How would you treat this patient?

4. Would you consider allowing this patient to have custody of her child again?

5. What is the prognosis?

6. Briefly, what do you know of suicide among schizophrenic patients?

Answers

Q1.

This woman is most likely suffering from florid schizophrenia with first rank symptoms such as thought disorder, believing others can read her thoughts, and auditory hallucinations commenting on her. She is also deluded and completely lacking in insight, and exhibits volitional and affective disturbance. There is no evidence from the patient, the relatives, or the social worker that she has recently taken drugs which might induce a psychosis and drug induced psychoses are in general more marked by florid perceptual disturbances than by disorders of volition, affect and thought. There is no evidence of marked depression at present. Her personality may of course also be immature.

Q2.

Schizophrenic patients, of course, may also get depressed and could respond to antidepressant therapy. In her previous admission she was under considerable stress caring for her infant, feeling isolated and very unsure about the future. This could have precipitated depression especially in a vulnerable personality, and there is no reason why she would not respond to antidepressants and/or supportive psychotherapy.

Q3.

It would probably be advisable to prescribe long acting intramuscular neuroleptic drugs rather than drugs to be taken a few times daily, as she may be unreliable with medication. Her injection could be given weekly or every two weeks by a community psychiatric nurse, and this would also ensure that a trained person was calling to the house at regular intervals who would observe her and liaise with the hospital. Ideally a mother and child unit would have been desirable to admit the patient and her child to in the first instance.

Q4.

Should this patient respond to treatment, there is no contraindication, provided there is good supervision in allowing her cutody of her child. It is probably better in general for a child to be cared for by a schizophrenic mother in remission than by a foster parent. Good supervision would include observation of her and her child at outpatients and by a social worker and a community psychiatric nurse at regular intervals. Of great help in a case like this is an interested relative, close neighbour or a nursery school supervisor who with the patient's agreement, has some insight into the problem and could help when community supportive facilities are at a low ebb at weekends or during holiday periods. The objective is to ensure that there is frequent observation without making the patient feel that she is hounded.

Q5.

The prognosis is probably poor. She is having frequent hospital admissions and is tending to become isolated socially and failing to cope in general. On the positive side there is no marked family history of schizophrenia, her presentation is usually very acute and there may be a depressive component to her symptoms. She has always been treated with oral medication and may be intramuscular neuroleptics will reduce her frequency of relapse and need for hospitalisation.

Q6.

There are variations from different centres on the suicide rate among schizophrenic patients, due probably to different subgroups studied. There is general agreement that the rate is high. It has been reported that 10 per cent of all schizophrenics kill themselves and that the rate is fifty times greater than for the general population. Chronic schizophrenic patients and those with persistent auditory hallucinations are thought to be at special risk.

Course and management

The patient was treated with modecate injections 40 mg weekly and responded to treatment after about three weeks. It was planned to give her trial leave in the near future and if successful to eventually give her custody of her child under multidisciplinary supervision, after discharge. She is to attend a day hospital twice weekly and in the first instance the child will be cared for by the grandparents and attend a nursery.

Further reading

Crow T J, Johnstone E C, Owen F 1979 Research on schizophrenia. In: Granville Grossman K (ed), Recent advances in clinical psychiatry 3, Churchill Livingstone, Edinburgh, London, New York p 2–11

Hogarty G E, Goldbert S C, Collaborative study group 1973 Drug and sociotherapy in the aftercare of schizophrenic patients. One year relapse rates. Arch Gen Psychiat 28: 54–64

Leff J P 1972 Maintenance therapy and schizophrenia. Brit J Hosp Med 8: 377

Leff J P, Hirsch S R, Gaind R, Rohde P D, Stevens B 1973 Life events and maintenance therapy in schizophrenic relapse. Brit J Psychiat 123: 659–660

Smith S M, Hanson R, Noble S 1973 Parents of battered babies: a controlled study. Brit Med J 4: 388–391

Wilkinson D G 1982 The suicide rate in schizophrenia. Brit J Psychiat 140: 138–141

CASE 39

A 40-year-old man is referred by his general practitioner because he is afraid to walk further than one hundred yards from his home. His mother had been diagnosed as suffering with agoraphobia, was treated with minor tranquillizers and attended psychiatric out-patients. Father had died about 10 years previously and he describes him as 'a strict disciplinarian, very Victorian'. He had a normal birth and childhood, without obvious neurotic traits. He was teased by his classmates for being 'skinny and tiny'. He was an average student. He left school at 16 and did odd jobs until he was conscripted at 18. He left the army at the age of 26 and did odd jobs in the building trade. From the age of 41 up to 43 (the year before admission) he worked as a porter but had to give that up when he could no longer get to his work due to agoraphobia. He divorced after five years of marriage and there were three children. He met his second wife in a pub. She was a divorcee with a 12 years old daughter and was 15 years older than him. The three of them live in a council flat and the relationship between them has fluctuated because she is intolerant of his agoraphobia. More recently she saw a programme on this subject on television and she is now more understanding. He describes himself as a tense anxious conscientious man who likes to keep himself neat and tidy. He was first treated in a psychiatric hospital in 1969 and diagnosed as an anxiety state in the setting of an inadequate personality. He had an operation for peptic ulcer in 1966 but is otherwise well medically. He admits to drinking to excess at times, as alcohol relieves his anxiety and he likes going to the pub with someone as this enables him to have a social outlet. At interview he is very neat and tidily dressed, very much on his guard, and does not appear relaxed during the interview. He denies feeling depressed but admits to being anxious and worried about his agoraphobia. There are no psychotic features evident. His agoraphobia has become particularly severe in the previous year for no apparent reason. He cannot drive his car, avoids public transport, shopping in supermarkets, or waiting in queues. He cannot relate the onset of his agoraphobia to any particular event. With increasing frequency he experiences panic attacks if he leaves home, thinks death is imminent and has marked palpitations. He is perplexed by his fears and realises they are irrational.

Questions

1. What is the commonest type of phobia seen in practice?

2. How can you distinguish between a primary anxiety state with phobic symptoms and a primary phobic disorder?

3. What other symptoms are frequently found in conjunction with phobias?

4. Which psychological mechanisms underlie phobic states?

5. How would you treat this patient?

6. Write a brief criticism of agoraphobia as a true phobia.

Answers

Q1.
Agoraphobia is the commonest phobia seen in psychiatric practice. The fear is frequently not confined solely to open places but may include fears of leaving the home travelling on buses, trains or lifts, of crowds and of confined spaces.

Q2.
It may be difficult to distinguish between the two conditions as phobic symptoms are common in anxious patients. Primary phobic disorders tend to pursue a long course with little fluctuation in symptoms, whereas in anxious patients variability with fluctuation in the secondary phobic symptoms may be noticed. In marked primary phobic states the irrational fears will completely dominate or paralyse the patient's daily activity. Affective disorder is commonly found with primary anxiety states — indeed it is doubtful if anxiety exists in pure culture, and depression is of course also found in conjunction with phobic states, so there may be considerable overlap in anxiety, affective, and phobic states.

Q3.
It is quite common to find phobias accompanied by symptoms of depression, depersonalisation, and of course panic attacks.

Q4.
Phobic. disorders commonly relate to a traumatic event e.g. after a car accident, the person may become fearful of travelling in cars. Conditioning and learning theory play important roles in initiating and maintaining the phobia. Anxiety ensures that the phobic situation is avoided and a form of operant conditioning is introduced.

Some phobias however do not appear to be associated with obvious trauma but appear to be more intimately related to affective change. Psychologically phobias are regarded as masks for unconscious anxiety related to neurotic repressions, the phobic situation comprises an avoidable representation of the genuinely feared object.

Q5.
Some form of behaviour therapy would probably be most appropriate in this case. A form of systematic desensitisation could be tried. The stimuli starting with the least are built up to the greatest anxiety provoking situation. The patient should be encouraged to practice relaxation at home. Mild anxiolytic drugs may sometimes be necessary to control a high level of 'free floating' anxiety. Alternatively the patient could be exposed quite quickly for a long period to a severe anxiety provoking stimulus (flooding). Some prefer this treatment for phobic anxiety states. Monoamine oxidase inhibitor drugs (M.A.O.I.'s) may help if there is marked associated depression.

Q6.
The concept of agoraphobia as a coherent clinical condition with well established features, has been criticised. It is found in many psychiatric conditions such as anxiety, affective disorders and obsessional states. It is a special feature of considerable intensity in many patients suffering from anxiety. In contrast to other specific phobias, the fear is broad and generalised and may not be confined solely or exclusively to open places but is frequently found to fragment into fears of crowds, public transport or noise. It is inclined to differ from other phobias in that on occasions it may be non-existent even in public places. It is suggested that agoraphobia is not a central feature of a phobic syndrome but a variable feature of patients with neurotic anxieties arising from a multitude of different origins. It has been suggested that to study the coping strategies of people with 'agoraphobia' may throw further light on the condition, and maybe there is a 'staying at home' rather than agoraphobic component in many anxiety states.

Course and management

The patient was treated with systematic desensitisation by a behavioural psychologist. He was brought to a day hospital by car and in company with the psychologist walked increasing distances from the day hospital. Eventually he walked in front of the therapist and out of the hospital grounds. He can now walk around the hospital if he is aware that the therapist is a hundred yards or so away. A milestone in the patient's subjective feeling of improvement was reached when he walked unaccompanied to a brick wall and informed the therapist that he kicked the wall with delight. He has been taught relaxation techniques and the panic attacks are becoming infrequent.

Further reading

Agias W S, Chapin N, Oliveau D C 1972 The natural history of phobia: course and prognosis. Arch Gen Psychiat 26: 315–317

Hallam R S 1978 Agoraphobia: a critical review of the concept. Brit J Psychiat 133: 314–319

Marks I M, Boulougouris J, Marset P 1971 Flooding versus desensitisation in phobic disorders. Brit J Psychiat 119: 353–375

Tyrer P, Candy J, Kelly D 1973 Phenelzine in phobic anxiety, a controlled trial. Psych Med 3: 120–124

CASE 40

A 32-year-old drug dependent man is admitted from a drug dependence outpatient clinic because he is stuporose and drowsy due to
excessive barbiturate intake. There is no history of drug dependence or psychiatric illness in the family background. His natural father
died when he was 10, mother remarried and he had a good relationship with his mother and stepfather as a child. There were no
pronounced childhood neurotic traits but he suffered with nocturnal enuresis up to the age of eight. He played truant frequently and
left school at the age of 15 without doing the 11+ examination, and
complained that when at school he 'got with the wrong crowd'. His
work record is poor, he held numerous jobs for short periods and
the longest time he worked was for one and half years as a carpenter. He is heterosexual, smokes about 20 cigarettes daily, but has
little interest in alcohol, has few interests or ambitions and a very
small circle of friends, most of whom are drug dependent. There
is no psychiatric illness antedating drug abuse and he is in good health
medically. The patient has taken unprescribed drugs for about 15
years. These included amphetamines, cannabis, physeptone, barbiturates, methaqualone and diazapam. He first used amphetamines, which he got from a 'friend'. and tried any drug he could
get. At the time of referral he is receiving maintenance therapy with
methadone 40 mg I.M. daily and is taking barbiturates, which he
gets on the black market. He suffered with a paranoid psychosis
10 years previously when he though people were following him and
he was treated in hospital for seven months. He took four inadvertent overdoses which needed medical treatment and one overdose with suicidal intent. He was arrested on three occasions once
for the possession of cannabis, once for malicious damage to his
mother's house and once for the possession of Barbidex after which
he was committed to Borstal for 18 months. At interview his nutritional and physical state is satisfactory, there are injection marks
on both ante-cubital fossae and he has widespread tattooing on hands
and forearms. He is living in a reception centre. He is sleepy and
drowsy, and finds difficulty in sitting up straight or answering questions. It is difficult to assess him mentally.

Questions

1. Give a short diagnostic formulation on this patient.

2. Distinguish between psychic and physical dependence on drugs.

3. Do you know of any ill effects of cannabis use?

4. What are your views of a drug maintenance treatment centre in the management of this patient?

5. What do you know of endorphins and encephalins?

6. Do you know of a physical or pharmacological explanation for the development of tolerance to a drug?

Answers

Q1.
This is a 32-year-old man probably psychologically and physically drug dependent, who has received treatment with Methadone maintenance therapy for about 10 years at an outpatient clinic. He is in reasonably good physical health, and has shown some psychopathic traits related to his drug habit, has little motivation and is probably a vulnerable inadequate personality. The prognosis is poor for the foreseeable future.

Q2.
Psychic dependence is present when a feeling of mental satisfaction and well being is only produced by, and dependent upon taking, a drug. Continuous or frequent administration of the drug is necessary to maintain this state, withdrawal of the drug will lead to mental disquiet and unease, so there is a compulsion to continue taking the drug. Physical dependence is present when the body has adapted itself physically and biochemically to the drug, so that when withdrawal occurs there is physiological disturbance which may include sweating, palpitations and vomiting. Psychic and physical dependence are closely related and their characteristics vary with individual drugs.

Q3.
Cannabis is a generic name for a variety of preparations and there is controversy concerning the ill effects of use. There are reports of severe intoxication resulting in gastro-enteritis and renal failure. Sometimes 'bad trips' are experienced, which appear to relate to the personality of the user and the setting in which he takes the drugs — there may be paranoid ideas, depression, and severe depersonalisation. Long term psychotic desorders have also been described. There is also considerable discussion on the production of an

'amotivational syndrome' in heavy cannabis users, characterised by lack of drive, effectiveness and spontaniety. The possibility of cannabis producing cerebral and chromosomal damage is also under discussion.

Q4.
The advantage of a drug maintenance programme for this patient is that it will provide him with a legitimate supply of his drug, reduce the likelihood or frequency of his incursions into the black market and of infringing the law to support his habit. It will also give an opportunity to medical and nursing personnel and social workers to supervise his general medical, psychological and social state, and hopefully reduce the physical complications resulting from use of non-sterile needles. Most addicts, of course, are poly-drug users, as this patient is. He moves in the drug 'scene' and most of his friends are addicts. He will probably continue to have crises and complications, some necessitating admission to hospital.

Q5.
Endorphins are endogenous opiate related peptides which were identified in the mid-1970s and the most commonly known is beta endorphin. They are found in the pituitary. They are thought to be functionally related to endogenous opiate neurotransmitters such as methionine and encaphalin, which are found usually in the limbic system. They are believed to co-ordinate and control sensory information concerned with emotion and pain. They appear to function as in-built opiates.

Q6.
The development of tolerance is a complex and poorly understood process. It is described as occuring at the hepatic and cellular levels. Enzyme induction to metabolise the drug is stimulated by increasing doses of the drug and at the cellular level there appears to be decreasing sensitivity to it's effects. Tolerance to morphine in particular can be viewed in the context of the encephalin system. Encephalins inhibit the release of neurotransmitters, such as acetylcholine from the presynaptic neurone. Morphine also has the same effect, so there is a compensatory biological response to exogenous opiates by induction of enzyme systems to produce more neurotransmitters, especially in neurones concerned with the transmission of emotion and pain. The end result is that more morphine will be required to inhibit the neurotransmitters and tolerance will develop to a specific dose.

Course and management

After admission to hospital he was supervised, and he did not require a formal barbiturate withdrawal schedule. He attended various social and rehabilitation programmes within the hospital. He showed no desire to withdraw from maintenance therapy and he was not pressurised to do so. He continued with methadone maintenance 40 mg I.M. daily, accommodation was found for him and he was discharged. with follow up at a drug maintenance clinic.

Further reading

Bewley T H 1970 An introduction to drug dependence. Brit J Hosp Med 4: 150–161

Clift A D 1972 Factors leading to dependence on hypnotic drugs. Brit Med J 3: 614–617

Davidson K 1981 Toxic psychosis. Brit J Hosp Med 26 (5): 530–537

Granville Grossman K 1979 Psychiatric aspects of cannabis use. In: Granville Grossman K (ed) Recent advances in clinical psychiatry 3, Churchill Livingstone, Edinburgh, London, p. 251–270

Thorley A 1979 Drug dependence. In: Hill, Murray. Thorley (eds) Essentials of postgraduate psychiatry, Academic Press, London, New York, p. 277–319

CASE 41

A 56-year-old woman, living in a patients' hostel, who initially appears to be without symtomatology but on close questioning claims that she is married to Jesus Christ and has 64 children by him is referred to a psychiatrist. Her father was a labourer, both parents died of natural causes, and she claims to have had a good relationship with them. She had a brother, and a younger sister, but they are both dead, and there is no history of psychiatric disturbance in the family. She describes herself as a warm, religious person, conscientious and hard working. Her previous medical history is irrelevant and she is in good physical health. There were no childhood neurotic traits. She attended school up to the age of 14 was an average scholar and had several jobs, mainly as a shop assistant, until her first psychiatric admission in 1950 when she remained in hospital for two years during which time she was diagnosed as schizophrenic and was leucotomised. She is heterosexual and although she has had a few boy friends she never married. After leaving hospital she lived with her mother for 20 years until the latter's death. She was admitted to hospital again in 1972 when she was depressed and unable to cope and has remained in a patients' hostel. During this period she has been treated with one course of E.C.T. and has received long acting neuroleptic intra-muscular preparations fortnightly. Overall she has remained generally well but was not considered capable of living independently outside of hospital. A period of training for a group home proved unsuccessful due to a clash of personality with other trainees. She has no particular desire to leave hospital at present and attends a day centre outside the hospital daily. At interview she is a pleasant co-operative lady, well adjusted to her environment, but appears to be lacking spontaneity and is without ambition. There is no cognitive defect and she will only talk about her delusion when questioned closely. There is no affective disturbance and she appears to be very happy with her life situation in the patients' hostel. She appears to be within the average range intellectually.

Questions

1. What is the diagnosis?

2. Does schizophrenia reach a 'burned out' phase?

3. What do you understand by an 'encapsulated delusion'?

4. What is your view on the psychopathology of delusion formation in schizophrenia?

5. Would you change the management of this patient?

6. What is the prognosis?

Answers

Q1.
This woman's history suggests she is schizophrenic, but it appears to be quiescent and at present she has a fixed encapsulated delusion which does not appear to be very disturbing to her. The schizophrenic process has left a marked deficit in her personality and she is of course grossly institutionalised and far too happy within the hospital setting.

Q2.
The term 'burned out schizophrenia' is frequently used in psychiatric practice, but there is little evidence to suggest that schizophrenia reaches an end state. Long term quiescent phases (smouldering phases) are common but the possibility of an acute flare up of symptoms can never be fully excluded.

Q3.
An encapsulated delusion is frequently found in quiescent schizophrenia. The patient is undisturbed by it and will only reveal it on close questioning. It is probably the end stage of a systematised delusional process and generally there are no other psychotic features evident.

Q4.
There are many views on delusion formation in schizophrenia. Often they can be seen essentially as attempts using normal principles of reason and experience to explain and understand basic misperceptions. It may be that schizophrenics are hyperaware and that too many percepts arrive in consciousness where they require interpretation and explanation. Delusion formation may be the schizophrenics way of interpreting and rationalising all these percepts. Delusions can, of course, occur in isolation (primary or autochthonous) are then not necessarily dependent on or secondary to hallucinations.

Q5.
Efforts at rehabilitating this woman should continue, or otherwise she may spend many more years in a hospital setting. She should again attend a rehabilitation assessment unit with a view to training in order to live either in an after-care hostel outside the hospital compound or in a group home and ideally she should work in a sheltered environment. She should continue with her anti-psychotic long acting intra-muscular neuroleptic at least until she has settled in the community and she should be followed up at outpatients and by a community psychiatric nurse. A social worker should also be assigned to her.

Q6.
The prognosis is probably poor. There will be difficulty in getting her to accept a life outside hospital especially as she has no close living relative to support her. The prognosis would improve if she found a group home with residents to whom she could relate. This would help fill a social gap in her life.

Course and management

The patient was discharged from hospital to a group home and attends an industrial therapy centre daily. She is followed up at outpatients.

Further reading

Bennett D H 1967 The management of schizophrenia. Brit J Hosp Med 7: 589–593

Frith C D 1979 Consciousness, information processing and schizophrenia. Brit J Psychiat 134: 225–238

Morgan R 1979 Conversations with chronic schizophrenic patients. Brit J Psychiat 134: 187–194

CASE 42

A 44-year-old man who attends a day hospital complains of feeling depressed and being persecuted by his workmates. He also has bouts of excessive drinking. His father was a coal miner who drank excessively and died of chronic bronchitis. The mother is alive and he has three sisters and one brother. There is no history of psychiatric illness in the family. He claims to have had a healthy happy childhood, attended school up to the age of 14, and was a reasonably good student. There were no childhood neurotic traits. He married at the age of 22, but separated after 15 years because the wife was unfaithful; there are two children both of whom live with the wife, whom he is in the process of divorcing. He spent 18 years in the merchant navy as an able-bodied seaman; in the last five years he has worked as an electrician. He claims to have done his job very well and that his employers refused to accept his resignation which he tendered prior to admission to the day hospital. He describes himself as quick tempered, hypersensitive and impulsive, a poor mixer, inclined to look on the black side of events and introverted. His past medical history is irrelevant but he has had many admissions to psychiatric hospitals for depression and alcoholism. He was admitted twice in 1974 and says, 'Once for treatment of alcoholism and once for depression'. There were several admissions for repeated overdoses in 1975. He was treated for depression in 1976 and had several admissions in 1977 also for repeated overdoses. He was treated as an outpatient with E.C.T. and antidepressants in 1979 and was admitted after there was no response to treatment. He was treated with imipramine 25 mg t.d.s. and showed slight improvement and was discharged after six weeks to attend a day hospital. He denies that alcohol is really a problem with him, and says he only drinks if he is feeling down and then does so episodically with drinking bouts only lasting for a couple of days. At interview he is dejected and tearful, there is psychomotor retardation, and he doesn't talk much. He admits to feeling depressed uniformly throughout the day, and there is no marked disturbance in appetite and sleep. He relates his depression to the misfortunes that have befallen him, such as his wife's infidelity and the persecution he receives from his workmates, whom he accuses of being hostile and of talking about him, criticising him and making life difficult for him. He does not know why they should behave in such a fashion. There are no suicidal feelings, but he had secluded himself in his flat before attending the day hospital. There is no disturbance of cognition.

Questions

1. What is the differential diagnosis?

2. What classifications of depression do you know of?

3. Discuss this man's belief that he is being persecuted.

4. How would you manage this case?

5. What is the likely prognosis?

6. Very briefly what do you know of new developments in anti-depressant medication?

Answers

Q1.

This man may be suffering with reactive depression in the setting of a hypersensitive personality and his episodic drinking could be secondary to his depression. The type of depression he is suffering from however, is unclear. He may have minimised his drinking problem and be suffering from alcoholism with secondary depression and paranoid delusions concerning the wife's infidelity and persecution from his workmates. An interview with the wife or some independent witness who knows him well would be of considerable help in clarifying the diagnosis, also reports from other hospitals would be very helpful.

Q2.

There are many systems of classification in depression and there is considerable confusion and on-going research in this field. Division into two categories of endogenous and reactive depression is probably the best known nomenclature for the disorder in Britain. Endogenous depression may arise out of the blue, is characterised by more severe depression, without reactivity, with guilt, and pessimism which may reach delusional intensity. There is disturbance in somatic function, appetite and libido may deteriorate and there may be marked sleep disturbance characterised by early morning waking. Reactive depression may be milder, and may be a response to stress of some kind, there may be difficulty in getting off to sleep and the depression may be worse in the evening. There is also a view that depression is a continuum with reactive at one pole and endogenous at the other. Depression has also been divided into unipolar where there is a history of depression alone, and bipolar where there is also a history of mania or hypomania. Depression has also been classified as type 'S' where there is a pronounced change in the functions of the hypothalmus with changes in appetite, sexual libido and sleep and type 'J' (Justified), justified by events. The terms primary and secondary affective disorder are being used increasingly in the United States depending on whether the depression has been preceded by any other psychiatric illness in the patient's life history. The existence of involutional melancholia as a distinct clinical entity seems to lack scientific support.

Q3.
This man's persecutory belief, which is delusional, may be explained in the setting of his depression, his drinking behaviour, or both. Delusions of persecution are common in the endogenous type of depression (though patients may accept them as justifiable punishment for their wickedness) and alcoholic patients frequently express delusions of infidelity on the part of the spouse. If the delusion is depressive in origin then it should decrease in intensity or disappear as his depression subsides. This patient's personality has been described as hypersensitive and he may readily take offence and harbour many beliefs of a persecutory nature concerning his spouse and colleagues, bordering on the delusional, even in the absence of depression or alcoholism.

Q4.
Further inquiries from relatives and friends and reports from other hospitals where he has been a patient should throw considerable light on the size of this patient's problem with depression and/or alcohol. This would also lead to a better understanding of the strengths and weaknesses of his personality. As far as possible he should be treated as an outpatient; he should have frequent outpatient appointments or see the doctor at the day hospital which he attends. He showed only marginal response in the past to tricyclic antidepressants and ECT, so it may be worthwhile prescribing a Monoamine Oxidase Inhibitor antidepressant for a therapeutic trial. Depending on the nature and extent of his problem with alcohol and his motivation, referral to an alcohol unit might be advisable. He should only be admitted to hospital if suicide becomes a very real danger.

Q5.
The prognosis for the foreseeable future is probably poor.

Q6.
Drug firms have expended considerable energy in developing new antidepressant preparations. There are now over 40 antidepressants both new and old listed. This reflects not only active promotion and indiscriminate prescribing but the relatively poor efficacy and high toxicity of some of these preparations. Research has shown that tricyclic antidepressants account for from 6 to 9 per cent of all overdose fatalities. In general, the claim for the newer antidepressants is that they are at least as effective as imipramine or amitriptyline while lacking their toxicity especially their cardiotoxicity. Along with 'tricyclic' drugs there are now one, two and four ring structured preparations with broadly similar properties. Among the better known newer antidepressants are included mianserin, nomifensine, viloxazine, maprotiline, flupenthixol and zimelidine dihydro-chloride. It is claimed for viloxazine that it is a non-sedative antidepressant virtually free of anticholinergic side-effects and safe when taken in an overdose. It is a tricyclic preparation. Mianserin is a tetracyclic with a biochemical effect different to tricyclics and has no influence on 5 hydroxy-tryptamine or noradrenaline uptake. It has no anticholingeric effects, is safe to use with antihypertensive agents. It has sedative properties and is relatively free of cardiotoxic effects. Maprotiline is a tetracyclic antidepressant but it has a side chain and a biochemical action similar to tricyclics. It militates against noradrenaline re-uptake. It is reputed to have a tranquilising effect and a rapid onset of action. Its anticholinergic effects are similar to the tricyclics and several deaths have followed overdose. Flupenthixol is a thioxanthine and an analogue of the phenothiazine fluphenazine. It was reported as being as effective as amitriptyline in depression and superior to it in anxiety. This effect has not yet been confirmed. Nomifensine is a tetrahydroisoquinoline and has a pharmacological profile similar to that of imipramine but with far less anticholinergic and cardiovascular effects. It inhibits both noradrenaline and dopamine re-uptake. It has been shown to be at least as effective as imipramine and amitriptyline, and has been widely used in the treatment of depression in the elderly. It must be administered in three divided doses as it has a short elimination half life, unlike most new antidepressants. It lacks a sedative effect. Zimeldine dihydrochloride is a recent addition to the group. Its molecular structure differs from tricyclic antidepressants and it acts by inhibiting the re-uptake of 5 H.T. It has a weak anticholinergic action and it is non-sedative. In

summary the newer antidepressants have not been proved to have greater efficacy over the old tricyclics but they are probably at least as effective. Trials have not been sufficiently large or well controlled to confirm their superiority over the well established drugs. It must be remembered that in most studies of antidepressants a placebo response of at least 30 per cent is present so that antidepressants as a whole are only between 20 per cent or 40 per cent better than placebos, and only between 1 in 3, or 1 in 5 patients are being pharmacologically helped by their medication. The newer drugs are probably not as effective as E.C.T.

Course and management

The patient continued to attend a day hospital where·he participated in group therapy, relaxation exercises and social activities. He still harboured persecutory ideas about his workmates but they were not as intense as before and alcohol did not appear to be a problem. He was treated with imipramine 50 mg t.d.s. with some alleviation of his depression.

Further reading

Gibson S, Becker J 1973 Changes in alcoholics self reported depression. Quart J Stud Alc 34: 829–836

Kendell R E 1976 The calssification of depression: a review of contemporary confusion. Brit J Psychiat 129: 15–28

King D J 1980 New developments in antidepressant medication — a review. Ir Med J 73 (10):

Paykel E S 1979 Reading about depression. Brit J psychiat 134: 211–213

Ritson B 1971 Personality and prognosis in alcoholism. Brit J Psychiat 118: 79–82

CASE 43

A 65-year-old man was referred to hospital by his general practitioner after he had apparently attempted suicide by jumping from
a low first floor window. He was born in Malta did well at school
and left at the age of 14. His father was a labourer, there was no
history of psychiatric illness in the family and he was the fourth of
seven siblings. He had a happy childhood and there were no childhood neurotic traits. He worked for short periods at tailoring and
as a hairdresser before joining the Royal Maltese Artillery before
the second war. During the war he saw quite a lot of action, refused
to accept a commission and was honourably discharged in 1945. He
worked as a labourer and then came to Britain in 1950 where he
has worked at many jobs including cooking and factory work. His
last job was as a toilet attendant for five years until he was sacked
'for failing to produce a doctor's certificate after being absent from
work'. He is heterosexual and was engaged but prevented from
marrying by the outbreak of war. Since then he has had three
relationships with women. He describes himself as a friendly man
who likes company; for many years he used to sing in public houses
and he believes he has a good tenor voice. Since the age of 14 he
has drunk alcohol, originally only wine, but for many years after
coming to Britain a half to three quarters of a bottle of whisky daily.
At present he claims to only take three or four pints of beer at
weekends. When he was drinking whisky he used to suffer with
'the shakes and the retches' but denies that he has any problem with
drinking now. He is a Roman Catholic and attends church regularly. For the last 13 years he has lived alone in a rented room and
complains of feeling very lonely and isolated there where he is on
bad terms with the Maltese landlord. He has a marked rhinophyma,
mild hypertension and minimal hepatic cirrhosis, but generally feels
quite fit physically. There is no previous psychiatric history. He has
been feeling more isolated for about three months, because he could
not go out to the pub as frequently as he used to, as alcohol has
become so costly and he was living on his old age pension. He used
to get many free drinks in pubs for singing, but thought his voice
was now fading. He believes the neighbours are talking about him
saying 'that fellow is a Maltese bastard he is always alone, he must
be a spy'. Also he hears voices of a very derogatory nature talking
about him when he is alone in his room and says he jumped out
of the window to escape the voices. He denies feeling suicidal as
he knew no serious harm would come to him as the jump from the
window was not very high. He did not injure himself. He is very

talkative during the interview and is generally pleasant and co-operative, but complains of feeling miserable, due mainly to his circumstances. If he is sent back to his rented room he threatens he will kill himself. He has a general feeling people are against him and he also still hears 'voices' but says they are worse when he is alone. Mentally he is quite lucid and there is no cognitive defects.

Questions

1. What is the likely diagnosis?

2. Would you describe this man as alcoholic?

3. What are the psychological disadvantages for this man in living in London?

4. What is the psychopathology of auditory hallucination formation in schizophrenia?

5. How would you manage this case?

Answers

Q1.

This man is probably suffering from paraphrenia. This is a condition usually regarded as a form of schizophrenia, characterised by auditory hallucinations of a derogatory kind but in which the personality is well preserved. However, this patient's history of excessive alcohol intake for many years and his loneliness and isolation living in an alien culture cannot be ignored as major contributory factors to his psychiatric symptomatology.

Q2.

We would need to know much more about this man's drinking history and habits before we could describe him as dependent on alcohol to such a degree that he is suffering physical, psychological or social impairment as a result. At present he claims that his drinking is restricted to a few pints of beer at weekends but his account may be unreliable in which case his paranoid symptomatology may be due to some degree to his alcohol intake. Rather than having alcohol dependence, he may be better described as having alcohol related disabilities, though we lack evidence for this. Apart from Wernicke's encephalopathy and Korsakoff's psychosis there are a wide spectrum of neuro-psychiatric consequences of alcohol consumption. The condition of alcoholic hallucinosis holds a central position. The patient hears voices usually of a derogatory nature; these may be associated with delusions of persecution, which may arise as explanations of the hallucinations. The chronic alcoholic may think that he is persecuted by all, that his spouse is unfaithful, and morbid jealousy is frequently encountered. This is sometimes described as alcoholic paranoia, and this patient has some evidence of this.

Q3.

There are obvious psychological disadvantages for this man living in a different culture. He is a single male in the lower socio-economic groups, English is not his first language and most of his relatives and friends he knew as a young man are in his home country. Loneliness and social isolation are a very distinct possibility for him and will exacerbate his paranoid feelings. However it is now accepted that not all immigrant groups have a high rate of mental illness and the emphasis is now on studying the different stresses, motivations, resources and patterns of settlement of individuals and groups.

Q4.

A psychodynamic hypothesis for hallucination formation in schizophrenia is that the ego disowns certain unpalatable thoughts or wishes which are then repressed and become unconscious. They may force their way back into consciousness, disguising their source by the mechanism of projection which makes them appear to come from outside the individual in the form of an external sensory perception. It has been claimed that three types of auditory hallucinations are diagnostic of schizophrenia. These are, voices which talk about the patient in the third person, those which make a running commentary on his actions and those that give the patient the impression that his own thoughts are spoken aloud (thought echo).

Q5.

Although this man's suicidal 'attempt' was probably more in the nature of a call for help than a serious effort at killing himself, he should nevertheless be admitted to hospital for psychiatric and social assessment. Early discharge should be planned as he may readily find the hospital life style socially acceptable, become institutionalised and be reluctant to leave. A tranquilliser at medium dosage, for example thioridazine 50 mg t.d.s. may help to control the anxiety emanating from his delusional beliefs and it is quite likely that with diversional occupational therapy and an acceptable social outlet the intensity of his delusions will decrease. Before discharge from hospital the social vacuum in his life style should be filled by arranging for him to attend a day centre, a day hospital, or a club. The question of whether he would like to be repatriated could also be discussed with him.

Course and management

He was admitted informally to hospital where the intensity of his paranoid feelings subsided considerably after about ten days. He attended occupational therapy and the social centre, and two weeks before discharge he attended the psychogeriatric day hospital which he now attends three days weekly, after he reluctantly left hospital. In the early days after discharge he tried to gain readmittance on two or three occasions but these attempts were resisted. He has now settled down well in the community attends the day hospital regularly, occasionally expresses paranoid feelings about staff, but is quite manageable, is well liked and runs errands for the more infirm day hospital patients. He did not wish to be repatriated. He is not on medication and still drinks at weekends. The prognosis is guarded.

Further reading

Cochrane R 1977 Mental illness in immigrants to England and Wales: an analysis of mental hospital admissions, 1971. Soc Psychiat 12: 25–35

Cox J L 1977 Aspects of transcultural psychiatry. Brit J Psychiat. 130: 211–221

Cox J L 1982 Medical management, culture and mental illness. Brit J Hosp Med 27(5): 533–537

Glatt M M 1974 Alcoholism. Brit J Hosp Med 2: 111–120

Kay D W K 1972 Schizophrenia and schizophrenia-like states in the elderly. Brit J Hosp Med 8: 369

CASE 44

As duty doctor you are called to see a chronic schizophrenic male patient in a large psychiatric hospital. The charge nurse complains that the patient has struck another patient and threatened to kill him because he wrongfully thinks the other is talking about him and criticizing him. The patient is 57-years-old and has spent 35 years in hospital since his first admission when he was diagnosed as suffering from schizophrenia. Both parents are dead, there are two brothers one of whom suffered with epilepsy. Both emigrated to Canada many years previously and he has no contact with his family. As far as can be ascertained there is no family history of psychiatric illness. His medical history is irrelevant but he has had difficulty in hearing for about 12 years and has a hearing aid which he does not use effectively and persistently. His father owned a small grocery shop and when originally admitted he described the patient as always backward at school and as having been rejected by the army 'because of nervousness'. From the age of 16 to 21 he intermittently worked at various types of labouring occupations but was always aloof and had few friends. Eventually he was incapable of holding down a job and was idle for about a year and a half before his admission to hospital. He was eventually referred to a psychiatrist after he refused to get out of bed. The psychiatrist found him unkempt, lying in bed, grinning and grimacing inanely. He was apathetic and withdrawn and had to be urged to reply to questions, he appeared to be listening to auditory hallucinations and smiled fatuously when asked about them. Overall he appeared insightless about his condition. Although his condition has fluctuated he was never considered well enough to be discharged from hospital after admission. Over the years he has been treated with deep insulin treatment, E.C.T. and drugs but has failed to respond to efforts at rehabilitation. His attendance at occupational therapy and industrial therapy has been erratic and unpredictable and he seems to lack the ability to persevere at work. There is no history of violent behaviour. At interview the patient is agitated and restless and his poor hearing makes the interview difficult. Apart from his belief that the patient he struck was talking about him and criticizing him, there are no acute overt psychotic features evident at present. He asserts 'I know the type of smile he had on his face, he was laughing at me and talking about me, the way to stop him is to slap him twice and then he's all right'. It is not possible to reason with him and he becomes truculent when it is tried. There is no cognitive impairment, he is not depressed and there is no clouding of consciousness. His present medication is pimozide 8 mg daily.

Questions

1. What is your formulation on this patient?

2. In which psychiatric conditions do you find paranoid symptoms?

3. What do you know of the psychopathology of paranoid states?

4. Write a brief criticism of the term 'thought disorder' as used in psychiatry.

5. How would you treat this man?

6. Which factors would influence your choice of antipsychotic drug for this patient?

7. What is the likely effect of poor hearing on this man's mental state?

8. Write a very brief criticism of the concept of schizophrenia.

9. What do you know of 'Labelling theory' and its relevance to psychiatric practice?

Answers

Q1.
A 57-year-old schizophrenic man with poor hearing, who has spent 35 years in hospital is at present exhibiting violent behaviour. This behaviour is associated with paranoid delusions about another patient whom he believes is talking about him and criticizing him. His violence is directed against this patient. There is no obvious reason for the onset of these acute symptoms as he was quiescent up to two days previously.

Q2.
Paranoid symptomatology may be found in a wide variety of psychiatric states. Delusions of a paranoid kind are found par excellence in association with hallucinations in paranoid schizophrenia. Paranoid delusions are also found in chronic alcoholism, especially delusions of infidelity on the part of the spouse. They may be observed in psychotic depression and in cerebral organic states especially delerious states. Patients with delirium tremens and those

who abuse or are dependent on amphetamines may also present with paranoid features. Personalities described as paranoid, that is those hypersensitive individuals who cannot accept even mild criticism may show a paranoid reaction to stress. Although paranoid symptomatology is widespread, its exact classification is controversial and some commentators hold the view that there is only a difference of degree between paranoid personalities, paranoia and paranoid schizophrenia.

Q3.

It is important to know that the word paranoid has always had a broader meaning in the rest of Europe than in Britain. In Europe it is generally accepted as meaning that one is subject to systematized delusions which as well as persecutory may also be hypochondriacal, grandiose, erotic or religious in content. In Britain paranoid means persecuted in a more limited sense to most psychiatrists. It is thought that the underlying mental mechanism involved in paranoid states is projection. The individual attributes hostile or aggressive attitudes to others which have arisen in the individual's psyche. Freud attributed the origin of these attitudes or impulses to failed repression of homosexual fixation. He did a classic psychoanalytical study of the autobiography of Daniel Paul Schreber who has been described as the most famous paranoid patient of all, and related his paranoid features to failed repression of homosexual tendencies. Paranoid states may evolve into grandiose states by a process of identification with the great 'persecuted' people of history such as Jesus Christ or Joan of Arc and frequently their identity is assumed.

Q4.

Although Bleuler gave pre-eminence to thought disorder in the diagnosis of schizophrenia, psychiatry has been plagued by the absence of agreement on its definition. There are a variety of competing hypotheses for a fundamental underlying deficit such as, loss of the abstract attitude, overinclusive thinking, defects in attention and the 'immediacy' hypothesis. Laboratory tests have not clarified the issue, and thought disorder does not appear to be confined to schizophrenia but may occasionally be observed in other psychiatric disorders such as mania and depression and in people who do not merit a psychiatric diagnosis. Confusion has arisen mainly because thought disorder is almost invariably subjectively observed from the patient's speech and language behaviour in the clinical situation. A substantial body of research suggests that thought and language are not perfectly correlated, and anyone can exert conscious control over his language behaviour and manipulate it to obscure or conceal his thoughts. Within the practice of clinical psychiatry thought disorder is synonymous with disorganised speech. Perhaps disorganised speech would be a more accurate term to use. However for the moment the term thought disorder is widely used and there are at least eighteen different types of language behaviours that are considered to reflect sub-types of thought disorder. Prominent among these types are poverty of speech (poverty of thought), derailment (loose associations), incoherence (word salad, jargon), clanging, neologisms, echolalia, blocking (interruption of a train of speech) and perseveration (persistent repetition of words, ideas or subjects). Some types of thought disorder considered important are found to occur so infrequently that they are thought to be of little diagnostic value, such as neologisms and blocking. Also of little diagnostic value for schizophrenia is the speech disorder characterised by derailment (loose associations) as it also occurs in mania. Some authors recommend that the practice of referring globally to thought disorder in psychiatric practice as if it were homogenous, should be avoided, and that the specific sub types occurring in particular patients should be noted in practice and research.

Q5.

It is important firstly to assess as far as possible what danger from violence the patient presents to others. There is no accurate way of doing this but the best guidelines at present are a history of serious violence and an age group under 50. This patient does not have any of these factors. After discussing with the patient the content of his delusional belief it should be possible to assess its intensity and whether his violent behaviour is also likely to be directed at others. Whether psychotropic medication is indicated and/or transfer to a more acute ward to provide greater supervision and remove him from the subject of his delusion should then also be more clear. If he is considered as not representing a danger to others then he should remain on the ward and may be tranquillisers such as chlorpromazine or thioridazine in moderate to large doses should be included in his treatment regime temporarily. Referral to an occupational or industrial therapy department to reduce his preoccupation with his delusion may be indicated.

Q6.

The choice of an antipsychotic drug for this patient would be influenced by considerations of the aspects of his presentation one aims to control and by the likelihood of particular preparations giving rise to side effects and by the anticipated duration of treatment. As the patient is restless, agitated and aggressive a drug with a marked sedative as well as antipsychotic effects would be desirable and the phenothiazine group of drugs would be considered. Chlorpromazine has pronounced sedative effects but may have moderate to severe anticholinergic effects and extrapyramidal side effects. Thioridazine has moderate sedative effects marked anticholinergic effects and minimal extrapyramidal side effects, and may be useful. Promazine may not be sufficiently active as an antipsychotic agent, and haloperidol may produce marked extrapyramidal symptoms particularly dystonic reactions and akathisia, perphenazine is less sedatory than chlorpromazine and has more frequent extrapyramidal side effects.

Sedatives and anxiolytics such as chlormethiazole and the benzodiazepine group of drugs could also be considered. Chlormethiazole may be beneficial in behavioural disturbances associated with psychotic illness but dependence may develop. It is cumulative and may result in drowsiness, dizziness and ataxia. It is probably advisable in this case to use oral rather than depot preparations as the patient may be experiencing a transient paranoid episode and side effects of oral preparations are more easily managed. A therapeutic trial of one of the above drugs therefore may be indicated starting with low dosages and increasing the dosage if required. The differences between the antipsychotic drugs are less important than the great variability in patient response and tolerance to secondary effects.

Q7.

The social and psychological problems associated with poor hearing are in need of further research. It has long been thought that hearing disorders may have a role in the genesis of paranoid states. The characteristics of deafness thought to be of importance are early age of onset, long duration and severity. Changes in psychological functioning takes place over a long period and the phenomena observed in sensory deprivation experiments do not appear to be relevent. It is reasonable to expect that the social isolation, communication disorders and disorders of attention and perception associated with prolonged poor hearing would have an ill effect on personality development and functioning and exacerbate the symptoms of this patient's underlying psychiatric illness. The precise relationship of disordered attention, perception and communication in the deaf to paranoid psychosis is still however quite speculative.

Q8.

Probably the most obvious and enduring criticism of the concept of schizophrenia is the lack of international agreement about what precisely is meant by it. The American concept is broader and more embracing than the British and European concept and the much criticised Russian concept lends itself according to some Western critics to abuse and misuse by the state to include within the diagnosis political dissidents. Szasz regards schizophrenia as a medical fiction invented by psychiatrists to serve their own and society's needs. Laing regards schizophrenia as the predictable response of an individual to a sick society. Others have criticised the labelling of individuals as schizophrenic as it may be a self fulfilling diagnosis inducing doctors, employers, society and friends to adopt an attitude toward the person which results in the person developing the symptoms of schizophrenia. The instability of the diagnosis over time and also in the clinical setting argues against it being a distinct single psychopathological entity. An analogy has been made between schizophrenia and use of the term 'a fever' by eighteenth century physicians who applied this to anyone with a raised temperature as if it were a distinct illness. It is possible that the word schizophrenia includes within it different clinical conditions as well, which will become apparent with further research and knowledge. It must be borne in mind however, that despite the above criticisms of the concept, there is much greater accuracy and high inter-rater reliability when a structured approach to the diagnosis is followed such as in the Present State Examination.

Q9.

'Labelling theory', also known as the 'Societal reaction perspective', is a sociological approach to the study of deviant behaviour. According to this theory, deviance is viewed as the end result of social processes involving an interaction between the person who commits the act and those appointed by society to respond to it and assign labels. In the context of this theory criticism has been levelled at psychiatrists as acting as the appointees of society to label individuals, without due regard to the clinical dictates which emphasis the importance of the personality, background and motivation of the individual. If this criticism were valid the violaters of social norms would be regarded as mentally disordered and those conforming to society as mentally stable. There is little evidence that in western psychiatry 'labelling theory' is of undue influence in the psychiatric diagnostic process.

Course and management

The patient was treated with chlorpromazine 50 mg six hourly for one week, when it was omitted. There were no further violent episodes.

Further reading

Andreasen N C 1979 Thought, language and communication disorders I. Clinical assessment — definition of terms and evaluation of their reliability. Arch Gen Psychiat 36(12): 1315–1325

Andreasen N C 1979 Thought, language and communication disorders II. Diagnostic significance, Arch Gen Psychiat 36(12): 1325–1330

Bean P 1979 Psychiatrists' assessments of mental illness: a comparison of some aspects of Thomas Scheff's approach to labelling theory. Brit J Psychiat 135: 122–128

Clare A W 1980 What is schizophrenia? In: Psychiatry in dissent — controversial issues in thought and practice, Tavistock Publications, London, p 120–168

Sim M, Gordon E B 1976 Basic Psychiatry, 3rd edn, Churchill Livingstone, Edinburgh, London. New York, p 178–179

Stevens J M 1982 Some psychological problems of acquired deafness. Brit J Psychiat 140: 453–456

CASE 45

A 37-year-old housewife with a history of asthma and recurrent eczema of the hands is referred from a dermatology clinic to psychiatric outpatients because of depression. She separated from her husband eight years previously, her two teenage children and her widowed mother are living with her. Her father was a cab driver and he died suddenly three years previously. There are three other siblings, she is the second youngest and there is no psychiatric history in the family. There is nothing remarkable about her early childhood years. She was an average student at school, and left at 16 without taking examinations. She worked at various jobs such as child minding, shop assisting and cleaning, up to the time her first child was born when she was 20 years old and had been married for approximately one year to a manual labourer. About one and a half years later her second child was born. She separated from and finally divorced her husband after about eight years of marriage because he abused alcohol and was violent to her and the children. She described herself as 'tense and anxious and inclined to worry a lot' and has few friends, she smokes moderately and doesn't drink. Her first bout of depression occurred about eight years ago after she was divorced, she was treated initially with tricyclic antidepressants and eventually received E.C.T. as an outpatient before recovering. Up to about six weeks previously she remained mentally well but in recent weeks has felt depressed, tired, lacks energy and drive, finds it difficult to perform her household tasks and get through the day. She cannot relate the onset of her depression to any particular stressful event, she has, however, a considerable number of problems. Her eczematous condition has worsened in the previous few weeks and has taken the form of acute cheiropompholyx. Her elder child lost his job as an apprentice joiner and she describes him as 'keeping bad company and needing a man to control him'. Also her mother is described as 'becoming difficult and makes a lot of demands on the family'. Apart from her history of asthma and eczema her past medical history is irrelevant, and her present medication is comprised of Betnovate cream and potassium permaganate soaks applied to her hands. Suicidal thoughts have never been entertained. Throughout the day she is uniformly depressed and cannot see any brightness in the future. Sleep and appetite do not appear to be greatly disturbed and there is no cognitive or perceptual disturbance.

Quesions

1. What is your formulation on this patient?

2. What do you know of current views on the influence of stress on the immune system?

3. What do you know of emotional disturbance in asthmatic children?

4. What effects may marital breakdown have on adolescent children?

5. Briefly comment on the statement 'Your mind is reflected in your skin'.

6. How would you treat this patient?

7. Summarise concisely the current consensus view on the use of E.C.T. in western psychiatry.

8. What do you understand by biofeedback techniques and do they have psychiatric applications?

9. Are mothers with young children psychiatrically vulnerable?

Answers

Q1.
This patient is suffering from a depression which has characteristics of both endogenous and reactive types, and maybe could be best described as atypical. The lack of energy, drive, and spontaneity, and the absence of a clear cut precipitating factor would suggest an endogenous type of illness. Also her history of a depression which responded to E.C.T. and tricylic antidepressants suggests, that she is again suffering from an endogenous depression. One cannot ignore, however, the considerable stresses she endures from worry about her health, her mother and son and of course she lacks the support of a husband in coping with her teenage children. These stresses could result in a reactive type of depression in a personality which she described as 'tense, anxious and inclined to worry a lot'. It is likely that she will again respond to appropriate treatment.

Q2.
Immunology is a rapidly advancing area of medicine and its inter-action with stress has come under scrutiny. The underlying hypoth-

esis of much of the research is that stress increases an organism's vulnerability to disease by means of an immuno-suppressive effect. The diseases intimately associated with immunological mechanisms such as malignancy, infections and auto-immune disease have received considerable attention. An intact normal neuroendocrine system is essential to the proper functioning of the immune system and of course the neuro-endocrine system is influenced by stress. The clinical literature underlines the importance of psychological factors in the precipitation and determination of the course of many physical illnesses. In the clinical and animal experimental fields it has been shown that stress alters cellular immune mechanisms. For example, bereavement is shown to be associated with depressed lymphocyte formation and in the experimental field antibody responses to antigens have been reduced by stress. It has also been demonstrated that lesions in the hypothalamus which is the controlling neuro-endocrine centre suppresses both humoural and cellular immunity. In studies done on patients with breast cancer and on patients with rheumatoid arthritis it has been possible to demonstrate adverse specific correlations between immunoglobulin levels and emotional states. Susceptibility to a wide variety of diseases may be influenced by stress and other psychological states but this must be viewed in the context of other influencing factors such as the genetic endowment and age of the individual.

Q3.

There is considerable literature on emotional disturbance in asthmatic children and much of it is concerned with the anxiety generated in striving for independence from parents. The anxiety triggers off an attack of asthma in the physically and psychologically predisposed child, and enables the child to influence and control the parents to some degree though his illness. However it also has a somewhat undesired effect in that it underlines his dependency needs on his parents. Physiological bronchospasm is common in the second and the third year of life and concurrent with this period, the child has to cope with the conflicting feelings of desire for autonomy from the parents and the fear and anxiety of separation. The psychological conflict may trigger off the physiological predisposition to asthma and result in an attack. Over a period of time, the child may respond to emotional conflic with an attack of asthma as a conditioned response long after the physiological factor has faded. The indication for psychiatric intervention is assessed not on the severity of the physical illness but on the degree to which the child's life circumstances generate emotional conflict.

Q4.

Adolescence may be a difficult time biologically and socially, and the support and understanding of well adjusted informed parents who share a stable marriage can be of considerable help to their maturing children. The adolescent experiences considerable intra-psychic conflict as he tries to control his aggression, regulate and understand his sexuality while he reconciles his desires for inde-pendence with the dependency needs of his family on him, and he on them. The pressures from peer groups on the individual to behave in a antisocial or delinquent manner are also great at this time. Marital breakdown is then but one of many pressures the adolescent may have to cope with and it may be a challenge the constitutionally unprepared may not be able to resolve. It has been shown that adolescent children of one parent families are especially vulnerable to delinquency and academic failure especially in the absence of the parent of the same sex. It has been found among boys in detention centres that those coming from homes where the parents have sep-arated or divorced were many times more commonly represented than those coming from homes where a parent had died or from 'normal' homes. It would appear that the disturbed marriage rather than the final loss or departure of one parent has the more del-eterious effect on the children. It must also be borne in mind that the family is a dynamic system, what effects one may effect all. The adolescent child may place insupportable stresses on a marriage which is already severely compromised and lead to its breakdown.

Q5.

The underlying premise in this statement is that the condition of one's skin is greatly influenced by one's psychological state. It is a common observation that an individual 'blushes' when emotion-ally embarrassed and may 'blanch' when submitted to sudden psy-chological shock, both effects being mediated through the autonomic nervous system. In many chronic skin disorders psychological fac-tors are accepted as associated influencing factors both in the onset and the course of the condition, via neuroendocrine control. Stress, neuroses, in general, affective disorders and anxiety states are fre-quently found in association with skin disorders. For example, affective disorders are thought to act as precipitating factors in such conditions as seborrhoeic dermatitis and acne vulgaris. Particular personality types who have difficulty in socialising and who have a high floating level of anxiety, are described as commonly to be found among individuals presenting with atopic dermatitis. It is also well known that although warts have a viral origin, psychological methods of treatment are frequently successful. Psychological sweating due to emotional disturbance occurs more commonly on the palms of the hands, the axillae and the soles of the feet and if the disturbance is chronic, rashes and bacterial and fungal infections of the skin may result. Urticaria is described as related to stressful life situations, and itching to tension and anxiety. Itching has been further described as having a pleasurable content comparable to an auto eortic experience or a masochistic function aimed at the infliction of pain to dissipate guilt. As many skin disorders are long term some of the associated psychological disturbances may be viewed as reactions to the stress of the disorders. Nevertheless to be aware of the possible psychological associations of skin disorders may be useful knowledge in their management.

Q6.

It would be worthwhile, in the first instance to see if she would respond to a tricyclic or tetracylic antidepressant over a period of three to four weeks. If she failed to respond to one particular antidepressant another could be substituted. Maybe a monoamine oxidase inhibiter would be more appropriate. Her symptomatology does not indicate clearly which is the more appropriate type of antidepressant. Some schools of practice recommend the use of combined tricyclic and monoamine oxidase inhibiter antidepressants in patients presenting like this, but despite claims of a very low incidence of side effects, this is still not accepted as orthodox practice. Concurrent with the exhibition of antidepressants there should be a socio-psychiatric assessment of the pressures on the patient to ascertain if there is a possibility of alleviating some of her problems. Maybe the patient's mother or teenage son have difficulties or problems which are adversely effecting the patient's health, or maybe the patient is but the 'iceberg' tip of a problem family, and a family approach is needed. Should the patient fail to respond to antidepressants and family or environmental manipulation then there should be no delay in introducing a course of E.C.T.

Q7.

The use of electro convulsive therapy in psychiatric treatment has situmulated interest, criticism, discussions, lobbying, legislation restricting its use, and research into its efficacy and mode of action. Its main use in western psychiatry is in the treatment of endogenous depression unresponsive to antidepressants. E.C.T. was widely used and a clinical impression of its efficacy was widespread before the introduction of double blind trials in the 1950's and 1960's. The overall finding of double blind trials was that E.C.T. was better than simulated E.C.T. More recent trials in the late 1970's and in 1980 and 1981 give somewhat conflicting findings. However the consensus view is that E.C.T. is a worthwhile treatment in endogenous depression when other treatments have failed. The efficacy of E.C.T. in schizophrenia is less clear, it may be helpful in acute schizophrenia with a depressive component but in chronic schizophrenia it is generally agreed that it is not of much value. Although E.C.T. is occasionally used in the treatment of mania there is no substantial evidence that it is superior to haloperidol, chlorpromazine or lithium in this condition. E.C.T. is a very safe treatment, but transient impairment of memory for a few weeks, is almost universal. However there is some evidence that long term impairment of memory can occur in some people. Many psychiatrists hold the view that E.C.T. was too liberally prescribed in the 1940's, 1950's and 1960's but this 'overprescription' may be indicative of the inadequacies of other forms of treatment and the lack of community and social support available at that time. Most western psychiatrists feel that E.C.T. is a very useful thereapeutic tool, but is not a first line treatment procedure and that further research to firmly establish its therapeutic efficacy is needed.

Q.8

Biofeedback technique could be described as based essentially on learning theory and particularly on operant conditioning. It can be defined as a technique by which an individual becomes aware at once of changes in bodily functions, so that eventually he can curtail these changes to his advantage. The advantage resulting acts as a tangible reward which maintains the change in bodily functions. Another theoretical view on the method of functioning is that biofeedback compliments the intricate endogenous feedback mechanisms necessary to homeostasis which when overloaded results in disease. The devices used are portable battery operated units with leads attached to the organ to be monitored such as muscle or skin. Information is fed back and processed and relayed to the subject in the form of visual display or auditorally. The patient with sufficient initiative and motivation for change, is trained in its use over a few sessions. It can be used in the treatment of tension headaches, anxiety states and migraine. For example in the treatment of anxiety states and tension headaches there is electro myographic feedback from the frontalis muscle by electrodes attached to the skin of the forehead. The patient is instructed to reduce the frequency of the electrical feedback, with subsequent reduction in muscle tension. This reduction in tension should become generalised. It is difficult at present to assess its place in therapy or its cost effectiveness. It would appear to have advantages in that the treatment can be used by 'normal' individuals as well as patients. After training individuals can control their own treatment and the equipment combined with the therapist can have a major placebo effect.

Q9.

There is considerable evidence that women with young children are psychiatrically vulnerable. It is reported that working class women with a child under six have a high risk of developing depression. There is also a high rate of depression in the mothers of pre school children especially three year olds. This may be related to the physical and emotional demands made by the child and to the mother's feeling of isolation. Poor housing conditions may also be contributory and women with children living in flats are more likely to visit their doctor with neurotic complaints than women living in houses.

Course and management

The patient was treated for three weeks with tricyclic antidepressants as an outpatient but she did not respond to treatment. As she was in a deep depression, she was then treated with a course of two E.C.T.'s weekly for three weeks and made a very good response to treatment. She continued to take tricyclic antidepressants for about six months and attended outpatients for about two months. The improvement in her affective state did not appear to benefit her skin condition.

Further reading

Kendell R E 1981 The present status of electroconvulsive therapy. Brit J Psychiat 139: 265–283

Kogeorgos J, Scott D F 1981 Biofeedback and its clinical applications. Brit J Hosp Med. 25(00): 601–606

Peterson E B, Evans J 1978 Psychiatric problems of adolescents. In: Forrest A D, Affleck J W, Zealley A K (eds) Companion to psychiatric studies (2nd edn) Churchill Livingstone, Edinburgh, London, New York, p 350–367

Richman N 1977 Behaviour problems in pre-school children: family and social factors. Brit J Psychiat. 131: 523–527

Rogers M P, Dubey D, Reich P 1979 The influence of the psyche and the brain on immunity and disease susceptibility: a critical review. Psychos Med 61(2): 147–164

Sim M, Gordon E B, 1976 Basic Psychiatry, 3rd edn, Chuchill Livingstone, Edinburgh, London, New York, p 137–140

Wolff S 1978 Psychiatric disorders in childhood. In: Forrest A D, Affleck J W, Zealley A K (eds) Companion to psychiatric studies, Churchill Livingstone, Edinburgh, London, New York, p 342

CASE 46

A 22-year-old woman is referred to psychiatric outpatients by her general practitioner. She complains of feeling depressed and also of being distressed because she believes her nose is too large. Her father is a solicitor and her mother is mainly occupied with housework. The patient has two younger male siblings. There is no history of psychiatric illness in the immediate family, but a second cousin committed suicide. Her early childhood was normal and she was an average student at school and left at 17 with three O levels. She then did a commercial secretarial course and has worked in this capacity in two jobs for the preceding four years. At present she is unemployed since she relinquished her job six weeks previously as she felt she could not 'keep up with it'. She experienced menarche at the age of 12, is heterosexual and has had a boy friend now for about 15 months, but has no plans for marriage. Her past medical history is irrelevant, and she describes herself as 'a reasonably good mixer, not particularly religious, interested in books and sport but at times inclined to be depressed and moody'. She shares a flat with a girl friend. There is a history of one admission to a psychiatric hospital three years previously for treatment of depression, which responded to antidepressants and E.C.T. During the previous six to seven weeks she has complained of lethargy, fatigue and insomnia with difficulty in getting off to sleep. She has also become very ruminative, thinking mainly on the apparent futility of life. Over the same period she has become increasingly subjectively depressed throughout the day and pre-occupied with her facial appearance, particularly the 'large' size of her nose. She is not sure whether worry about her facial appearance antedated her depression. With increasing depression she has developed some features of obsessional behaviour such as checking and re-checking at work and a tendency to wash her hands more frequently than would be necessary. She was prescribed tricyclic antidepressants by her general practitioner over a period of about four weeks but they were ineffective. Thoughts of suicide have entered her mind, but she thinks she would not kill herself 'mainly out of concern for the upset and worry it would cause my parents'. There is no exacerbation of her symptoms premenstrually or during menstruation. Her appetite is also impaired and she has lost about a stone and a half in weight over about two months. To the interviewer her facial appearance is unremarkable. She speaks in a low monotonous voice, her mood appears depressed, there is marked psychomotor retardation and little facial expression. There is no paranoid symptomatology present and apart from her belief about her facial appearance there are no delusions and no perceptual disturbances.

Questions

1. What is your formulation on this patient?

2. What is your concept of dysmorphophobia?

3. Is there a prognostic distinction between delusional and non delusional depression?

4. Have you heard of any vulnerability factors predisposing to depression in working class women?

5. What is the management and prognosis for this patient?

6. Comment briefly on the statement 'The only certainty in psychiatric practice is uncertainty'.

7. Very briefly what in your view are the characteristics of a good psychiatrist?

8. What is the 'Capgras syndrome'?

Answers

Q1.
There are at least two main diagnostic hypotheses which could be formulated on this patient. Firstly, this patient is probably suffering from an endogenous type of depression, with depression of mood, anergia, loss of initiative, drive and appetite and suicidal ruminations, and psychomotor retardation. Her worry about her facial appearance could be described as secondary dsymorphophobia and her obsessional behaviour would also be regarded as secondary to her depression. Secondly, an alternative hypothesis is that worry about her facial appearance has precipitated a reactive type of depression in a vulnerable personality. There is, however, little evidence for describing her personality as vulnerable beyond her description of herself as 'at times inclined to be depressed and moody'. There is also no clear cut evidence that the worry about

her facial appearance antedated her depression. The response of her previous depression to antidepressants and E.C.T. would suggest that her present illness is of the endogenous type. The possibility that we are witnessing the start of a schizophrenic illness cannot be totally excluded as depression of mood and worry about facial appearance are not uncommonly found in schizophrenia.

Q2.

Dysmorphophobia could be described as a subjective belief of some physical deformity noticeable to others, although the physical appearance is within normal limits, and as a result of the belief the subject is tense and anxious and may seek plastic surgery. It may be a symptom complex of neuroses in general depression, schizophrenia, and personality disorder. It is regarded by some as an ominous symptom and represents a break-down of the ego boundaries with distortion of the body image, which is hypothesised to occur in schizophrenia. Long term studies comparing groups of patients requesting rhinoplasty for aesthetic reasons with those requesting it following diseases or trauma show a significant increase of patients with neuroses and schizophrenia in the former group. However, the vast majority of patients requesting surgery for aesthetic reasons are psychiatrically normal. Maybe dysmorphophobia assumes its poor prognostic role only in the presence of other psychiatric features.

Q3.

In the pre E.C.T. period of psychiatric treatment it was noted that most inpatients suffering with endogenous depression eventually improved. The small number who did not recover was almost totally comprised of patients with associated delusions. With the introduction of E.C.T. both groups were equally responsive to treatment. Some observers state that delusional depressives are unresponsive to tricyclic antidepressants and thatthe presence or absence of delusions in depression should be considered as an important criterion in the classification of depressive disorders and for the choice of treatment.

Q4.

It is reported that women who have lost their mother before 11-years-old, have three or four children at home under the age of 14, are not working outside the home situation and have not a confiding marital relationship are particularly vulnerable to depression. Separation from the father before 17 may also be a vulnerability factor. It is unknown what role personality plays in relation to these factors, and they may not be specific to depression alone.

Q5.
In the first instance it is worthwhile reassuring the patient about her facial appearance. Another tricyclic antidepressant could be prescribed as a therapeutic trial on the assumption that the patient is suffering from endogenous depression and she should be seen frequently (weekly if possible) at outpatients for supportive psychotherapy. If over a period of three weeks there is no marked response to treatment then a course of outpatient E.C.T. should be considered. The danger of suicide does not appear to be pronounced so she could continue as an outpatient. If she is unresponsive to antidepressants plus E.C.T., then the original diagnosis may have to be reviewed. The possibility that the patient is suffering from a predominately reactive type of depression, a personality disorder or is exhibiting signs of incipient schizophrenia would have to be considered. Admission to hospital for further observation, for psychometric assessment and a trial of alternative treatment such as the use of neuroleptic medication, or more intensive psychotherapy may be appropriate. The prognosis is uncertain.

Q6.
This statement underlines the observation that psychiatry is probably the least exact scientifically of all the medical specialities. The complexity of its subject matter readily explains its inexactness. Patterns of mental functioning and human behaviour are determined by many complex and conflicting influences, genetic, social, educational and cultural. The challenge in the individual patient may consist in unravelling and assessing the importance of each factor in contributing to his abnormal mental functioning and behaviour, and then to influence benignly the adverse factors. Consensus opinion on a psychiatric definition of normality which could be used as a measure of abnormality under changing circumstances and settings, is lacking, and unlikely to be obtainable in the foreseeable future. The brain is generally accepted as the centre of biological malfunction in many psychiatric states, especially the functional and affective disorders, and of course direct research on the living organ is technically difficult and may be ethically prohibited. Although psychiatry has many similarities with general medicine of the mid nineteenth century, which was mainly concerned with clinical observation and description, considerable advances have been made. The advent of antidepressants and neuro-

leptics have in conjunction with improved social support, rev-
olutionised the treatment of depression and schizophrenia. There
has been a dramatic fall in the populations in large psychiatric
hospitals and structured interviewing techniques and international
cross cultural studies have contributed considerably to exact diagnosis. Although uncertainty exists in the individual clinical case on
the most appropriate diagnosis and on the form of treatment most
likely to be successful, in general there is much more agreement
on diagnosis and treatment. The good psychiatrist should be aware
of the fallibilities and be flexible and willing to review diagnosis
and treatment.

Q7.

It has been customary to assess the qualities of a psychiatrist by
enquiring how effective he is in the treatment of patients. This is
particularly true when there is lay assessment of him. His colleagues, however, may also use other criteria such as research and
teaching ability or administrative talent. The good psychiatrist must
frequently ask himself during his professional life what effect a
particular activity has on the patients immediately under his care
and on patients in general. If the activity has a beneficial effect and
makes proper use of resources then it is something in which the
good psychiatrist can get involved. Apart from immediate care of
patients, activities such as administration, teaching and research
aimed at preventing psychiatric illness and developing better treatment facilities and methods of treatment can justifiably claim some
of his time. On the personal level he should have a good knowledge of his speciality, avoid espousing any particular school of
thought to the exclusion of others, be eclectic and able to adapt
his treatment to the changing needs of his patients, and to be kind
to patients while avoiding undue emotional involvement. He should
be able to orchestrate the talents of para medical personnel in
multidisciplinary harmony, while remaining aware of the fallibility
of his knowledge and not feel that his final responsibility for the
patient's welfare has been threatened. Finally he should be ready
to accept ongoing responsibility to care for patients who do not
respond adequately to treatment.

Q8.

The 'Capgras syndrome', first described by Capgras and Reboul —
Lachaux in 1923 is a delusional state in which the individual
believes that a double has assumed the identity of a closely related
person. It is rare, women are more often afflicted than men, and

the patients exhibiting it have a clear sensorium. The most frequently associated psychosis is paranoid schizophrenia and less often a schizoaffective, affective or organic psychosis is seen. The supposed substitutes are more often multiple than single and the number may increase with time. The delusion may be short lived, recurrent or of long duration. Treatment is directed at the related psychosis.

Course and management

The patient was treated with another tricyclic antidepressant as an outpatient but did not show any improvement after a three week period. She then had a course of eight E.C.T.s as an outpatient after which she showed some improvement, her depression was less pronounced and the anxiety about her appearance was less. She did not return to work within a period of six months and continued to attend outpatients regularly.

Further reading

Felstein I 1982 Psychiatrist or surgeon — who should treat the cosmetic problem patient? Psychiatry in practice. (June): 23–24

Gibson M, Connolly F H 1978 Dysmorphophobia — a long term study. Brit J Psychiat 132: 568–570

Hill D 1978 The qualities of a good psychiatrist. Brit J Psychiat 133: 97–105

Kantor S J, Glassman A H 1977 Delusional depressions: natural history and response to treatment. Brit J Psychiat 131: 351–360

Roy A 1978 Vulnerability factors and depression in women. Brit J Psychiat 133: 106–110

Todd J, Dewhurst K, Wallis G 1981 The syndrome of Capgras. Brit J Psychiat 139: 319–327

CASE 47

A 34-year-old woman is referred to psychiatric outpatients by her general practitioner for treatment of depression. Her father died about 15 years previously, he was a compositor, the mother is still alive, there is one older sibling and there is no history of psychiatric illness in the family. There is no history of childhood neurotic traits, she was a good student at school and left grammer school at the age of 16 with three 'O' levels. After leaving school she had various occupations, including clerical work, dental receptionist and telephonist. She married at the age of 24. The husband was five years older than she and she knew him for two years before marriage. He worked as a sub-manager in a lorry hire service and she describes him as an easy going ineffectual personality. There are three children, one aged eight, one seven and one three. She describes herself as 'strong-willed, quick tempered, sociable and a little anti-authoritarian'. She smokes moderately and rarely drinks alcohol, has not worked outside the home for four years and rarely goes out with her husband. She watches television for long periods in the evenings. There is a long history of depression dating back to when she suffered with puerperal depression after the birth of her first child. On that occasion she took an overdose of anti-depressants and was treated as an inpatient with antidepressants and E.C.T. and recovered. Two years later she had another depressive illness which again needed hospitalisation and E.C.T. and this was also accompanied by an overdose of drugs. For the preceding three years she remained 'fairly well but never 100 per cent'. Her medical history is unremarkable. Over the preceding two months she has become increasingly depressed, has lost interest in life, her appetite is poor and she has lost about a stone and a half in weight. She has remained sexually frigid since the birth of her first child, eight years previously. This is causing some friction in her marriage, which in turn is making her feel more miserable. Another symptom she complains of is insomnia — she has difficulty in getting off to sleep when she awakens in the early morning. Throughout the last month she has entertained suicidal feelings and at present is thinking of taking another overdose which she says 'would finish it all off'. The onset of her illness cannot be related to any clear-cut stress. At interview she is sullen and withdrawn, plainly dressed and not wearing make-up. She admits to feeling depressed and suicidal. There are no perceptual disturbances evident, and she will only speak when spoken to. Her husband who accompanies her, confirms that she has deteriorated mentally in the preceding two months, has become anergic, depressed and is lacking spontaneity and drive, and says that she has lost considerable weight. He confirms her statement on sexual frigidity and asserts 'we have come to live with it' and says that he makes no particular demands or criticisms of her.

Questions

1. What is your formulation on this patient?

2. How great in general is the problem of suicide?

3. How do you assess the likelihood of this patient again attempting suicide?

4. What is your concept of female sexual frigidity?

5. Comment very briefly on the statement — 'It is a mistaken view that Freud regarded the sexual problems as basically psychologically determined'.

6. Which psychological disturbances may be observed in the puerperium?

7. How would you manage this patient?

8. Do you know of any obstetric or social factors related to psychiatric admission in the puerperium?

9. What do you know of delayed onset of maternal affection after childbirth?

Answers

Q1.
This patient is suffering from a depressive illness which is predominately endogenous in type. It is characterised by subjective depression of mood, lack of energy, initiative and drive, disturbance of sleep and appetite and the presence of suicidal thoughts. There is no clear-cut environmental stress, apart from a long standing generalised sexual frigidity which is causing some dysharmony in the marital relationship, although her husband claims to be tolerant.

There is a history of at least two previous depressive illnesses occurring over an eight year period. The first occurred during the puerperium after her first child, the more recent illness about five years ago. On each occasion she responded well to hospitalisation and treatment with antidepressants and E.C.T. When psychiatrically well she is a reasonably good personality.

Q2.

Suicide presents the psychiatrist with a considerable problem. Apart from the deaths occurring in the natural course of the organic psychoses and the dementias, it is the greatest cause of death encountered in psychiatric practice. It is estimated that approximately 1 per cent of all deaths in Britain are caused by suicide. It is a problem in the young and old. In the 15 to 34 years age group it is the fourth most common cause of death, and suicide is also common among the elderly. The rate varies from country to country. The more prosperous countries without a religious taboo on suicide have higher rates than less prosperous countries, where the religious tenets of the populace forbid it. The low figures in Catholic countries, however, may be due to some degree to a certain reluctance on the part of coroners to bring in verdicts which would stigmatise the deceased and the relatives.

Q3.

Although there is no accurate method of predicting the likelihood of a suicidal attempt there are general and individual criteria which are helpful. In general, suicides rates are higher for the single, for males, for widows, for those with few or no children, for migrants, for those lacking an occupation and for those without religious belief. People in social classes I and II especially those in the professions have high rates. On the individual basis the number and seriousness of previous attempts is a good direct indicator. The presence of a depressive illness or an illness which is beginning to respond to antidepressant treatment and where there is a return of initiative and spontaneity is associated with increased risk. Suicide has a high rate among alcoholics. An overt suicidal threat can never be ignored and the ready availability of the means of carrying out the threat must always be heeded in assessing the individual risk. On the basis of these criteria the risk of suicide for this patient would appear to be considerable.

Q4.

Female sexual frigidity can be defined as a relative or absolute loss of capacity for genital sensual pleasure or of any pleasurable emotional experience normally associated with genital pleasure. In the lay mind and sometimes in the professional one also, the condition is misinterpreted as total and irremediable. The condition may be short term or long term and there is always a loss of the ability to achieve orgasm. It may be due to many causes. Common among these are a fear of pregnancy, lack of privacy, faulty technique on the part of the partner, such as the use of a withdrawal technique for contraception, inadequate sexual foreplay, depression, anxiety and marital dysharmony. There is frequently a temporary period of frigidity following childbirth. If there is a problem with sexual orientation, then frigidity may also be found, but usually one can achieve orgasm by masturbation and may express disgust at the thought of sexual intercourse. Treatment consists in identifying the causative factor or factors, removing them, discussing the problem with both partners and emphasising the temporary nature of the problem. Frigidity unresponsive to these approaches can be influenced by behaviour therapy.

Q5.

Contrary to many popular views this statement is probably true. Freud is among the most misinterpreted writers in history and difficulty and argument about what precisely he said and, more importantly what he meant, has flourished over the years. The 'Three Essays on the Theory of Sexuality' which first appeared in 1906 was his most important work on the sexual disorders. He makes it clear in his fourth edition of this book that his theory of sex was the most biological of all the concerns of psychoanalysis and that his aim was to find out how much could be guessed about the biology of human sexuality by psychological research. He concluded that underlying the perversions 'there is indeed something congenital', but went on to say that this 'something' was inborn in all humanity although it varied in intensity. He viewed sexual disorders on a continuum ranging from the most severe abnormalities to normality. He helped to remove the absolute divide. Sexual abnormalities were viewed as modifications of the normal sexual life. He sought to explain the development of the sexual instincts in relation to the developing psyche, and to state that when the sexual instinct failed to gain ascendency at a particular time a sexual perversion would result. While instincts were common to all he regarded their strengths and weaknesses as primarily constitutionally determined. He commented that the parts of his teachings which border on biology including his theory of sexuality continued to be misunderstood even by his followers.

Q6.

Psychiatric disorders occur more commonly in the three months after delivery than in any three month period in the two years preceding or the two years after. Temporary emotional disturbances are common in the puerperium. Transient depression sometimes called 'postpartum blues' can affect over 50 per cent of women, and usually does not need psychiatric intervention. A small minority of cases may go on to develop true clinical depression which will need treatment. The term puerperal psychosis has a typical onset about three or four days after delivery and it may be applied to a psychosis occurring up to one year past partum. It may be ushered in with clouding of consciousness. There is probably no clear cut reason for regarding it as different from a psychosis occurring outside the puerperium. It has an incidence of two to three women per one thousand deliveries and usually presents with a depressive or schizophrenic picture, but there may be some overlap. Paranoid hypochondriacal and nihilistic ideas may accompany the depression. The patient with the schizophrenic psychosis will present with volitional disturbance, auditory hallucinations and thought disorder. It is sometimes necessary to separate the mother and baby because of the risk of injury to the infant. The response to antidepressants or phenothiazines as appropriate and E.C.T. when necessary is usually good. Infrequently patients present with a neurotic disorder post partum, this may occur in vulnerable personalities and take the form of an anxiety or phobic state. Anxiety about the ability to cope with a baby may be seen in primiparae but this does not need psychiatric intervention and can be resolved by nursing advice and reassurance.

Q7.

This patient should be admitted to hospital for observation and treatment, because she presents a considerable suicidal risk. She could be treated with another antidepressant in hospital, but if she failed to respond she should receive a course of E.C.T. It is likely that she would respond to this. Once her depression has subsided, the cause and severity of her frigidity should be investigated. There may be some improvement in this concurrently with improvement in her depression. The subject should be discussed with the husband and wife and any apparent cause should be removed. The dynamics of the marital situation should also be explored. If no improvement can be effected then referral to a therapist specialising in the treatment of sexual dysfunction should be considered. This patient's frigidity is of such long duration that referral to a therapist specialising in sexual problems may be needed.

Q8.
It has been shown that first pregnancies are more commonly associated with puerperal psychosis and psychiatric admission than subsequent pregnancies. If a woman is unfortunate to suffer with puerperal psychosis in her first pregnancy, she may avoid subsequent pregnancies. Still it is thought, however, that first pregnancies are inherently more likely to be followed by puerperal psychosis and psychiatric admission. There also appears to be an increased risk of psychiatric admission attached to being single, widowed, divorced or separated. Delivery by caesarian section is also associated with psychiatric admission during the puerperium. Of course, women who have had one puerperal psychosis are at high risk of having another which may need psychiatric hospitalisation. Having the first baby, while single, by caesarian section could be regarded as a very stressful life event, capable of causing severe psychiatric illness. As the relative risk of psychotic illness after childbirth is considerably higher than that associated with other life events, other mechanisms such as hormonal and metabolic changes associated with childbirth may also play a role in the etiology of puerperal psychosis.

Q9.
Many mothers experience delayed onset of affection for their babies. This has been regarded as a normal variant by some observers and as an advantage by others, as bonding is deferred until the baby's survival is assured. Up to 40 per cent of primiparae and 25 per cent of multiparae have been reported as emotionally indifferent when holding their baby for the first time. Difficult labours, medication administered to the mother during labour and the use of intrusive obstetric procedures have been investigated as possible causative factors. Most mothers develop affection for their babies within a week and no long term adverse effects are seen.

Course and management

The patient was admitted to hospital and treated with a course of six E.C.T.s over a period of three weeks and received concurrently amitriptyline 50 mg t.d.s. She improved considerably and was discharged after a period of one month's hospitalisation. During her period in hospital the sexual problem was discussed weekly with the patient and her husband and both gained considerable insight. After discharge it was planned for the patient to attend outpatients accompanied by her husband, so that progress could be monitored. She continued to take antidepressants.

Further reading

Hoenig J 1976 Sigmund Freud's views on the sexual disorders in historical perspective. Brit J Psychiat 129: 193–199

Kendell R E, Rennie D, Clarke J A, Dean C 1981 The social and obstetric correlates of psychiatric admission in the puerperium. Psych Med 2(2): 341–350

Mordecai Robson K, Kumar R 1980 Delayed onset of maternal affection after childbirth. Brit J Psychiat 136: 347–353

Pierce D W 1981 Predictive validation of a suicide intent scale: a five year follow up. Brit J Psychiat 139: 391–396

Spencer E 1974 Psychosexual problems in women. Medicine (First series) 30: 1793–1796

CASE 48

An elderly couple is seen on a domiciliary consultation at the request
of their general practitioner. The wife, who is 60-year-old, complains that her 69-year-old husband has become doubly incontinent
over the preceding 9–10 months, is very confused and tends to wander
out of the house and get lost and has to be brought back by the police.
He has difficulty in finding his way around the home and cannot
make his way back from the neighbouring street. She is receiving
diazepam from her doctor and relates her anxiety intimately to the
worry and anxiety attached to caring for her husband and continues
'unless something is done I shall have a nervous breakdown'. She
has no psychiatric history, and says she does not wish to be separated from the husband but realises that she can no longer cope with
him. Their accommodation is comprised of a two bedroom mai-
sonette which is clean and carpeted. There is one daughter, married
and living in Australia. A district nurse visits once weekly and the
couple are living on their old age pensions and also get financial
assistance from their daughter. The husband has what is described
as 'bilateral progressive hearing loss' and refuses to wear a hearing
aid. He sits rather motionless and is inaccessible to questioning. His
wife says that he was well psychiatrically up to about 20 months
previously when he was admitted to the local hospital for investigation of epilepsy and a brain tumour was diagnosed. He was discharged from hospital and she claims that she was informed that
'nothing could be done about the tumour', but he was reviewed
regularly at outpatients. Since then he has gradually deteriorated
and become more confused and difficult to manage, although he no
longer has epileptic fits. A medical report from the hospital states
that the patient has a right parietal tumour which is displacing the
normal cerebral structure across the midline and measures about
4 cm in diameter. It is thought to be a glioma and surgery or
radiotherapy is not indicated. On examination he is able to walk in
an ataxic slow way with the help of a stick, he has a left sided hemi-
plegia, and there is no papilloedema. His present medication is
carbamazepine 100 mg t.d.s. A recent review at outpatients showed
the tumour to have increased considerably in size.

Questions

1. What is your formulation on this couple?

2. What is meant by the term 'normal pressure hydrocephalus'?

3. What is the dysmnesic syndrome?

4. Which cerebral sites serve the function of memory?

5. Do you know of any theories on the process of memory?

6. Would you briefly classify the important causes of dementia.

7. What would be the likely psychiatric sequelae if this tumour were sited mainly in the frontal lobes?

8. How would you manage this couple?

Answers

Q1.
Although it is difficult to fully assess the old gentleman psychiatrically due to his hearing loss, from the account of his wife, he is most likely suffering with a deteriorating confusional state intimately associated with his enlarging cerebral tumour. He was mentally lucid up to the time of onset of epilepsy associated with his growing tumour. There appears to be concurrent increase in his degree of confusion and in the size of his neoplasm, and it is possible that he may be experiencing increasing intracranial pressure; papilloedema is, however, absent. His confusion could be related to normal pressure hydrocephalus which may sometimes be found with cerebral tumours. The physical and psychiatric outlook for him is, of course, extremely poor and terminal care will very soon be necessary. The wife's anxiety appears intimately related to the stress, fatigue and worry attached to caring for her husband and difficulty in accepting that hospitalisation may be unavoidable.

Q2.
Normal pressure hydrocephalus may commonly present with dementia. The abnormal accumulation of cerebrospinal fluid is confined mainly to the ventricular cavities. It may be associated with a history of meningitis, head injury, subarachnoid heamorrhage or cerebral tumour. The patient may present with a slowly progressive dementia, urinary incontinence and disturbance of gait. Pneumo-

encephalography may show extreme dilatation of the ventricles with little or no air observed over the hemispheres and no other direct evidence of hydrocephalus. The introduction of an atrioventricular shunt may have a very beneficial effect on the patient and greatly ameliorate his symptoms.

Q3.

In its pure form the dysmnesic syndrome (Korsakoff syndrome) is characterised by impairment or loss of recent memory and preservation of immediate recall, remote memory and other cognitive functions. For example a patient can repeat a series of letters or numbers but if his attention lapses momentarily, he fails to recall what he repeated. The preservation of other cognitive function enables him to converse rationally on familiar topics. He will fail to recall events which occurred since the onset of his illness, but this failure will be masked by confabulation, into which the patient has no insight, but he will speak with assurance and conviction. The condition results from bilateral damage to the limbic system and the mamilliary bodies. The commonest cause of the condition is chronic alcoholism (often preceded by an episode of Wernicke's encephalopathy). It may occur in any condition associated with acute thiamine deficiency. Occasionally a transient dysmnesic syndrome may be observed during the recovery phase from severe head injury or from a subarachnoid haemorrhage. It is important to note that the dysmnesic syndrome is rarely seen in pure form as pathological processes involving the limbic system will frequently involve other cerebral sites, resulting in partial syndromes or syndrome complexes. As the limbic system is important in maintaining normal affect, disturbances of affect are also noted and these may take the form of apathy, lack of emotional response and sometimes of euphoria. The prognosis depends on the cause. In alcoholics, progressive brain damage may result in the syndrome slowly merging into dementia.

Q4.

For many years, memory was regarded as primarily a function of the hippocampus and certain mid-brain and thalamic sites. Recent research has endeavoured to identify specific areas of the brain serving different types of memory. For example memory has been subdivided into 'association', 'abstract' and 'representational' types. Association memory (stimulus response memory) will survive gross reduction in the mass of the brain and will actually be improved by lesions in the hippocampus. It will survive total removal of the neocortex. Its precise cerebral site has not been identified but it is believed to be subcortical. Representational memory, which serves the function of preserving images of previous events and personal experiences is served jointly by the hippocampus and the frontal cortex. Abstract memory which perceives the meaning of objects and events separate from mere recall of the events is regarded as largely a function of the neocortex. For example damage to cortical areas — temporal, parietal or occipital-serving abstract memory may result in object and facial agnosia. Much of the knowledge on cerebral memory sites has been derived from animal experiments and there are limitations in extrapolating memory research findings from animal to man, with his highly developed neocortex and language function.

Q5.

In discussions on the process of memory it is usual to divide it into short-term and long-term. These are now generally regarded as two components rather than continuous phases of memory. There is considerable agreement that a reverberating electrical circuit, of short duration, is the basic mechanism involved in serving short-term memory. Certain highly specialised neurones perform this function. There is much more disagreement on the process of long-term memory, and especially on the precise nature of the permanent memory trace. It has not been established that it is molecular, or that changes in coding occurs in nucleic acids, or that the synthesis of new proteins or peptides is involved, although these have been the main theories put forward and the lines of research followed. Some workers have stated that the retention of a trace is associated with a permanent change in the structure of RNA and others have noted an associated synthesis of an additional protein or peptide. It has also been proposed that the permanent trace in long-term memory is facilitated by neuronal cell change particularly the growth of bigger and better synapses. As each cortical neurone may have up to 10 000 synapses on its surface, and the brain may have 14 ms 10^9 cells, there would be the potential to code all the experiences of a lifetime. All the above observations may be valid, rather than contradictory views of an on-going process of long-term memory retention, however, the field is still rather speculative.

Q6.

The important causes of dementia, like the causes of many clinical conditions can be classified into infective, metabolic, traumatic, degenerative, familial, neoplastic and vascular causes. Among the infective causes the most prominent are, of course, meningitis, encephalitis, and meningovascular syphilis. Creutzfeldt-Jacob's disease is now regarded as having a slow virus origin. The metabolic causes are numerous and the most prominent are chronic alcoholism, vitamin B 12 deficiency, myxoedema, hypopituitarism, heavy metal poisoning and of course cerebral anoxia. Traumatic causes of dementia include of course road traffic accidents and birth injuries. Trauma is a relatively common cause of brain injury, especially in males up to the age of 45. The degenerative conditions of course include the senile and presenile dementias, and paralysis agitans. Among the familial conditions the commonest by far is Hungtington's chorea, and progressive myoclonic epilepsy could be included in this category also. A cerebral tumour may result in dementia and it is the most likely explanation for this patient's confusion, but any tumour metastasising to the brain, (and among the most prominent is carcinoma of the bronchus), may result in dementia. Vascular causes of dementia are numerous and any condition leading to sudden gross cerebral infarction or small multi-infarcts over a period of time may cause it. Included in this category are cerebral haemorrhage, blood or fat embolism or cerebral thrombosis. A subdural haematoma is a relatively common vascular cause of confusion which when recognised may be readily treatable.

Q7.

It is likely that the patient would suffer from the 'frontal lobe syndrome'. This is characterised mainly by a change in personality. The patient becomes less aware of social inhibitions and less sensitive to the feelings of others; he may undress or urinate in public. He ignores the consequences of his actions, and may eat, drink and smoke to excess. Euphoria or apathy may also be observed. The patient may become brash, over-talkative, self-assertive, restless and irritable. When apathy is evident, he will be withdrawn and aloof and will only respond monosyllabically to questioning. Cognitive function may be well preserved. The pure frontal lobe syndrome will only be seen when the pathology is limited to the frontal lobes such as is seen in trauma or very localised tumours. Modified features of the syndrome may be observable in more diffuse cerebral pathology such as in the early stage of Pick's disease (fronto temporal atrophy) but in the later stages the symptomatology may be overshadowed by other aspects of this condition, such as dementia.

Q8.

The old gentleman should be re-admitted to hospital as he may now need terminal care, or at least more care than his wife can give him. If he is again discharged from hospital, he should not go home, as a nursing home or terminal care home is more appropriate. It is likely that the wife will improve considerably psychiatrically when the burden and anxiety of caring for her husband is removed. It is probably advisable to allow the wife to continue to take diazepam temporarily and see her at outpatients as she may need help in coping with guilt feelings related to the hospitalisation of her husband. Guilt feelings could become acute should the husband die shortly after admission.

Course and management

The husband was admitted to hospital for long term care and the wife improved considerably after the husband's admission. She joined a relative support group where she discussed her feelings openly and she needed no further medication.

Further reading

Kiloh L G 1975 Psychiatric disturbances of organic origin. Medicine (Second series) 10: 460–468

Kopelman M 1981 Psychological aspects of neurology. Brit J Hosp Med 26: 367–379

Norton A 1981 Old men forget. Brit Med J 283: 1201–1202

CASE 49

A junior doctor is called to see a 27-year-old female patient on a psychiatric ward. She is a chronic schizophrenic and is described by the ward sister as 'becoming more deluded over the preceding two to three weeks'. There is a long history of psychiatric illness and she had her first admission to hospital at the age of 17. She presented in an acute psychotic manner, with perceptual, affective and behavioural disturbance. Over the years she has been treated with phenothiazines and has been discharged from hospital for short periods. She has failed to get a job or function in the community for very long, and efforts at rehabilitation have been unsuccessful. Both parents are alive and there are three other siblings, the patient is the second youngest. The patient was a full term normal delivery, there were no childhood neurotic traits and she was an average student at school. Shortly after leaving she had her first psychiatric hospitalisation. She became withdrawn, deluded, refused to get out of bed and was aggressive and violent towards the parents. Over the years the relationship with her parents has become very strained; they do not welcome her home as the mother's physical health is poor and she cannot cope with the patient. The patient has long entertained the belief that a famous film star is in love with her, and intends to marry her. This delusion has become more acute in recent weeks and she believes he was recently sending her messages when he appeared on television. Also she has become paranoid about the staff and accuses them of trying to make life difficult for her. Recently she tends to spend long periods in the bathroom washing herself and also is described as 'spending hours in front of the mirror putting on make-up'. At interview the patient is insightless and is unresponsive to an appeal to reason. She is auditorally hallucinated, voices command her to get some of her teeth removed and to lose a lot of weight. Voices also comment on her appearance and talk about her in the third person. She appears to engage in irrational conversation at times, as if she was responding to auditory hallucinations. At other times she appears withdrawn and looks as if she is depressed. She attends occupational therapy daily but is described there as 'very slow and wastes a lot of time attending to her appearance'. There is no obvious precipitating factor to her present symptomatology but she did have a row with her parents about two weeks previously and came back early from week-end leave. Her present medication is comprised of fluphenazine 100 mg I.M. every two weeks, chlorpromazine 50 mg orally six hourly and orphenadrine 50 mg six hourly. This has not been changed in over a year as her symptoms were considered well controlled on this regime.

Questions

1. What is your formulation on this patient?

2. What is De-Clerérambault's syndrome?

3. Which causative family or parental theories of schizophrenia do you know of?

4. What do you understand by the term 'pseudo hallucinations'?

5. What is the role of a 'token economy' programme in the treatment of chronic hospitalised schizophrenic patients?

6. How would you briefly assess the prognostic indices for this patient?

7. How would you manage this patient?

8. What do you understand by the term 'reactive psychoses'?

Answers

Q1.
This patient is most probably experiencing an acute exacerbation of her schizophrenic illness. The cause of her relapse is unknown, as it frequently is in schizophrenia, but the row with her parents may have been of some importance. There was no change in medication or personal circumstances which might have contributed to exacerbation of her symptoms. Her delusion that a famous film star is in love with her and intends to marry her is suggestive of 'psychose passionelle' (De Clérambault's syndrome). It is likely that the acute phase of her condition will ameliorate with time, however, as she is very disturbed at present her medication and management needs to be reviewed.

Q2.
De Clérambault's syndrome is characterised by a delusional belief, usually in a woman, that a famous man or a man of much higher social status, with whom she has had no contact, is in love with her. The person selected may be a film star, a top executive, a politician or a public figure. The delusion is held with great intensity, has a sudden onset, and the object of the delusion is always believed to have made the initial advances. She will deny all obstacles to this love such as marital state or distance. The existence of this condition as a definite clear cut syndrome is not fully established. It has been observed in the setting of frank schizophrenic symptoms and in paranoid psychoses. Patients with these delusions may bring chaos into the lives of their 'loved ones' by pestering them with letters, telegrams and telephone calls over a period of years. The underlying psychopathology is complex and ill understood but efforts to explain it on the basis of erotomania, have been attempted. It is also suggested that it may be a form of narcissism projected onto another or a defence mechanism aimed at denial of unconscious homo-erotic trends by substitution of a delusional heterosexual attachment. De Clérambault himself described it as essentially a form of sexual pride which leads on to desire and eventually hope. The prognosis is generally poor, with a tendency towards chronicity.

Q3.
There are five prominent theories on the family as a cause of schizophrenia. Probably the best known theory is that of R.D. Laing. It is a sociopolitical model in which schizophrenia could be viewed as a social label for deviance, a healthy reaction to a sick society, or as resulting from disturbed parent child relationships. Although his views are productive of speculation and discussion, they are difficult to research. The theory of Lidz is that there are two types of family distortion (marital skew and marital schism) which result in abnormal parental roles and communication and that this in turn leads to schizophrenia in the offspring. Bateson's double bind theory is well known. This is essentially based on a form of abnormal family communication, whereby the child receives contradictory messages. He is placed in a paradoxical situation, does not know how to think or respond appropriately and so withdraws or behaves ambiguously. The fourth theory is that of Wynne. He postulates that the families of schizophrenic individuals exhibit 'psuedomutuality'. They give a spurious impression of mutuality of approach and thought but underlying this is very poor communication or consensus. Over a period the child develops unrealistic patterns of thought and behaviour in response to this. The term the 'schizo-

phrenogenic' mother was born of efforts to describe characteristics peculiar to the mothers of schizophrenic individuals. The mothers have been described as overprotective in a passive way towards male patients and in an aggressive way towards females, and the characteristics are more likely to be observed in the mothers of process shizophrenics. It is important to know that none of these theories have been validated by carefully controlled investigations and these would be difficult to carry out. They arose from the subjective clinical observation of their proposers and most likely are not specific to the parents of schizophrenics. Evidence is still missing to support the view that specific parental or indeed familial characteristics operative during the formative years of the child increased the likelihood of it developing schizophrenia. This does not mean of course that these familial and parental characteristics may not precipitate or exacerbate latent or existing schizophrenia.

Q4.

The term 'pseudo hallucinations' is confusing and many of the standard psychiatric textbooks contain no reference to it. There is at present no consensus view on what precisely is meant by it. Part of the explanation for this may be the inability of language to grapple clearly with all the complexities of psychiatric phenomena, and the differing ways in which the word 'hallucination' is used. 'Pseudo hallucinations' have been described by various authors as either hallucinations in which insight is maintained, or as hallucinations not having the qualities of a percept in being related to external space, but coming from within in the form say of an inner voice, or merely as representatives of a specific type of imagery. There is considerable doubt then about the precise meaning of the term and also of course about its clinical usefulness. They are said to be observed, depending on the definition used, in states of clouded consciousness such as may be observed in those under the influence of hallucinatory drugs or experiencing sensory deprivation, or in hypnagogic states. In these conditions there is likely to be at least a quick return of insight. 'Pseudo hallucinations' in the form of 'inner voices' may be observed in depressive psychoses and obsessional states. Provided one defines precisely what one means by the term 'pseudo hallucination' it may be of some help in differentiating the above conditions from schizophrenia.

Q5.

The 'token economy' is a form of behaviour therapy which was introduced in the late 1960s. It has been used considerably in the treatment of chronic hospitalised schizophrenic patients who have deteriorated socially and behaviourally. It is essentially a form of operant conditioning in which 'tokens' or rewards are given to patients for the performance of specific desirable tasks such as getting up on time, making his bed, arriving at therapy punctually and regularly, and looking after his personal hygiene. With tokens the patient can purchase certain privileges such as attendance at various recreational or diversional activities, or permission to increase his television viewing time. The precise value of each token's purchasing power and the number of tokens which can be issued for the performance of particular tasks is made explicit to the patient. Particularly desirable types of behaviour can be re-inforced considerably by increasing their token value. There are many reports of the success of the 'token economy' in improving the behaviour of schizophrenic patients, to the degree that they may be considered suitable for discharge. However, the relapse rate may be high when patients are discharged as they may have difficulty in generalising to other situations.

Q6.

The diagnosis of schizophrenia has been established for this patient over many years. In this condition prognostic indices can be divided into pre-morbid and morbid groups, and each can be further divided into good and bad. The good pre-morbid indices comprise no family history of schizophrenia, a good work record, stable personality, late age of onset and a supportive family background. The bad pre-morbid indices, of course, include the converse of these. The good morbid indices comprise prominent affective symptoms, acute onset and a known precipitating cause, the presence of catatonic symptoms, few first rank symptoms and the preservation of initiative and drive. Bad morbid indices will, of course, include the converse of these. This patient's prognosis based on these criteria is poor, she has never worked and has a poor relationship with her family. There is no evidence that the onset was acute or obviously related to a cause, but was insidious. She has exhibited several first rank symptoms, and has never been catatonic. She is unrealistic and lacking in initiative and drive. The most ominous prognostic factor for this patient, of course, is her record of having spent most of the preceding 10 or 11 years in hospital despite efforts at rehabilitation, which strongly suggests that she has process schizophrenia.

Q7.

The patient may be experiencing a temporary acute relapse which will be self-limiting and minimal intervention may be necessary. Her symptoms have been reasonably well controlled on her present medication for over a year and it should not be altered readily. The patient should remain under observation and be seen daily by the doctor. Should no improvement occur after a further week or should the patient become violent to the staff as a result of her paranoid feelings, then her medication should be reviewed. The fluphenazine could remain unchanged, but the chlorpromazine could be increased to 75 mg to 100 mg or more six hourly until her symptoms are controlled. It may be necessary to try a series of drugs and different dosages until the patient responds. If evidence of a concurrent depression becomes apparent then E.C.T. may be the treatment of choice. Once she has improved, and maintained her improvement for one to two months then it would be worthwhile trying to reduce her medication to its original maintenance level.

Q8.
Although the term 'reactive psychosis' looks like a contradiction in terms, it was approved by the World Health Organisation for inclusion in the eight revision of the International Classification of Diseases. Most frequent reference to it is found in the Scandinavian literature. The psychosis is described as occurring in a particular personality type at a particular time in response to a clear cut environmental stress, traumatic experience or adverse life situation. The psychosis is intelligible in the context of the severity of the traumatic event reacting with the adverse personality traits of the patient. Also the context of the psychosis reflects and is coloured by the traumatic experience and as soon as it is neutralised or reversed, the psychosis terminates. The patient remains insightless as distinct from a patient with a neurotic reaction and frequently presents with paranoid symptomatology. The onset is usually acute, and the duration is brief ranging from a few weeks to a few months. It is a difficult diagnosis to make with certainty as other types of psychoses such as functional and organic must be ruled out, and one must declare with a degree of certainty that the stressful event was of such magnitude that a psychosis would not have occurred without it. The diagnosis is not in common use in British psychiatry.

Course and management

The patient's medication was changed by increasing the dose of chlorpromazine to 100 mg six hourly. Within a week the patient was considerably improved. She still entertained her delusions but was less disturbed by them. It was planned to return to the patient's original treatment regime as soon as possible.

Further reading

Cooper F E 1974 Diagnosis and treatment of schizophrenia. Medicine (First series) 30: 1744–1751

Enoch M D, Trethowan W H 1979 De Clérambault's syndrome. In: Uncommon psychiatric syndromes, 2nd edn, John Wright and Sons Ltd, Bristol, p 15–35

Fairburn C G 1981 Schizophrenia — a psychiatry seminar. Hospital Update 7(11): 1115–1127

Hare E H 1973 A short note on pseudo-hallucinations. Brit J Psychiat 122(569): 469–476

McCreadie R G, Main C J, Dunlop R A 1978 Token economy, pimozide and chronic schizophrenia. Brit J Psychiat 133: 179–181

Retterstøl N 1975 Paranoid psychoses. Medicine (Second series) 12: 528–535

CASE 50

A man of about 45–50-years of age is brought to casualty by the superintendent of a night shelter for 'down and outs' and is seen by the duty psychiatrist. He presented there the previous day when he was brought along by another resident who found him in the street. There is no history available from the patient, he is disorientated for time, place and person, and knows nothing of current affairs. He knows his name, but otherwise recent memory is grossly impaired and remote memory is also very poor, and he is in clear consciousness. On psychiatric assessment he is incapable of retaining new information, and there is no evidence of depression. His affect appears appropriate but may possibly be a little blunted. He is co-operative, answers questions to the best of his ability, and makes no attempt at confabulation. In appearance he is unkempt and untidy, but a recent hair cut is suggestive of recent residence in one or more institutions. Apart from blisters on both feet and flea marks on his skin, and a slight ataxic gait, physical examination is negative.

Questions

1. What is your differential diagnosis?

2. Very briefly compare Creutzfeldt-Jakob and Pick's pre-senile dementias.

3. What are the characteristics of hysterical amnesia?

4. Is there a relationship between Munchausen's syndrome and conversion hysteria?

5. How would you manage this patient?

6. Is there a role for 'reality orientation' in the management of this patient?

7. Is there a place for the use of cholinergic agents in the treatment of this patient?

Answers

Q1.

There are a few diagnostic possibilities to be considered with this patient, all relating to his main symptoms of cognitive impairment. Prominent among the diagnostic considerations is pre-senile dementia. In clear consciousness he has gross cognitive impairment and a global amnesia characterised by gross disturbance of recent and remote memory, inability to retain new information and disorientation for time, place and person. There is also social and personality deterioration. Admission from a reception centre for 'down and outs' suggests that he has drifted down the social scale and that his mental state has been deteriorating over a period of time. There is no evidence that he suffered recent head injury or cerebral damage that might account for his condition. His amnesia has not the characteristics of hysteria. The possibility that he is suffering from a Korsakoff type of dysmnesic syndrome is unlikely, in that his memory disturbance is global, there is no confabulation or effort to mask it, his sense of personal identity is not retained and there is no evidence of alcoholism. The possibility that he is suffering from a neurological or psychiatric form of Munchausen's syndrome is remote, as his presentation would be uncommon and he did not seek hospitalisation. Transient global amnesia secondary to vertebro-basilar artery insufficiency to the medial aspects of both temporal lobes is also unlikely as this is acute in onset, may only last a few hours, and remote memory is usually well preserved. Full neurological and physical investigation and observation over a period of time in hospital should greatly clarify the diagnosis. One of the numerous treatable or untreatable causes of confusion may be unearthed.

Q2.

Creutzfeldt-Jakob disease is an uncommon disorder believed to be due to a transmissable virus. It affects both sexes equally and has an onset when the patient is in the 40s or 50s. Widespread cerebral atrophy involving cortical and sub-cortical areas is seen. Involvement of the cerebellum spinal cord and brain stem is frequently noted. Neurological disorders are prominent with impairment of speech, cerebellar ataxia tremor, spasticity and various motor signs. Myoclonic jerks with a characteristic E.E.G. pattern help to establish the diagnosis. If the pathological process involves the anterior horn cells there is related muscle weakness and atrophy. Associated with these signs is a rapidly increasing dementia. There is no treatment. Death usually occurs within a year but may occur within months of onset.

Pick's disease is also an uncommon disease and is of unknown etiology and there may be a constitutional predisposition. It affects females twice as frequently as males, and has its onset in the 50s or early 60s. Cerebral atrophy in frontal and temporal lobes is seen, and neurofibrillary tangles and plaques are characteristically absent. In the early stages personality changes are seen characterised by deterioration in social behaviour and loss of restraint. The patient is fatuous and loses initiative, drive and insight. Neurological signs are less marked than in Creutzfeldt-Jakob disease and may be absent but dysphasia and incontinence may be present. The personality deterioration is soon followed by dementia. The E.E.G. is normal, in contrast to Creutzfeldt-Jakob disease. The diagnosis of Pick's disease is frequently only established by post mortem examination of the brain. There is no curative treatment, and ongoing nursing care eventually becomes necessary.

Q3.

Hysterical amnesia may be characterised by loss of memory for a specific circumsribed episode and usually the patient is seen in casualty, fully conscious, complaining that he does not know who he is or where he comes from. Cognitive function is otherwise fully intact and the patient can recall learned information that does not have emotional or personal connotations. This discrepancy in cognitive function may be stark and will be a considerable aid to diagnosis. As distinct from organic cognitive impairments there will be no obvious social and personality deterioration. The amnesia may be seen in the setting of a hysterical fugue state. The patient may wander off from his home or neighbourhood to avoid some unpleasant or threatening situation such as an interview by the police. Some days later he may find himself a long distance from home, having slept rough for a few nights and wondering what happened. Hysterical amnesias commonly subside within a few days but difficulty in recalling precipitating causes may persist. There is a tendency for these amnesias to occur in patients with a previous history of head injury and loss of consciousness. There may be an underlying psychiatric illness such as depression, or the condition may be seen as a component of a primary hysterical neurosis, or in association with underlying physical disease. It is ill advised to readily accept primary hysterical neurosis as the definitive diagnosis in amnesia.

Q4.

Munchausen's syndrome is related to other psychiatric conditions in some respects. Among the conditions with which it is thought to share some features are hypochondriasis, malingering, pseudologia fantastica and, of course, conversion hysteria. Although there is considerable agreement on the psychopathology of hysteria, such as the presence of an underlying pervasive anxiety, the somatic symbolic representation of hidden intrapsychic conflict, sick role playing and the achievement of primary gain, there is little agreement on the psychopathology of Munchausen's syndrome. The early environment of these patients is nearly always disadvantageous and it is thought that they may be conditioned to using symptoms to gain attention. This may be the method by which a grudge against the medical profession for some act subjectively judged to be harmful, finds expression. It is also thought to represent the expression of a desire for a change of sex, with surgical operations symbolising castration and for the expiation of deep seated feelings of guilt by surgically inflicted suffering. Although there are some psychopathological similarities with hysteria, such as somatisation and attention seeking, in general it would appear that the psychopathology is different. Clinically the condition may be distinguished from hysteria by the patient exhibiting remarkable medical knowledge, by appearing in casualty rather than at the general practitioner's surgery, and by the presence of an intense overt desire for hospitalisation, investigation and surgery. Examination of the patient's clothing may also show that he has hospital marked garments and his pockets may contain sharp intruments such as pins, or pieces of glass which have been used to produce bleeding. Physical examination may reveal numerous laparotomy scars. If questioned about a psychiatric history they may express mistrust of psychiatrists and trust in surgeons and physicians. Enquiries may reveal that the patient is well known in other hospitals or to previous casualty officers.

Q5.

This patient should be admitted to hospital for full physical and psychiatric assessment, and although the patient is only aged 45 to 50 a psychogeriatric assessment ward may be the most appropriate setting. The patient will then be assured of full physical assessment. Neurological investigations will include skull X-ray, E.E.G. and brain scan to exclude possible treatable conditions such as cerebral neoplasm or subdural haematoma. Investigations will also centre on the endocrine and nutritional state of the patient.

Liver function tests may throw light on whether the patient's mental state could be related to alcohol abuse or dependence. Should the patient's confusion persist and no treatable cause for it is found then psychometric testing to accurately assess the degree of confusion is indicated. If longterm psychiatric care is inevitable then the patient should be placed on a ward where the staff is engaged in ongoing orientation therapy, to maximise his potential.

Q6.
'Reality orientation' (R.O.) is a technique used in the rehabilitation of patients with memory loss, episodic confusion and time, place and person disorientation. It has been developed and used mainly in North America and is divided into two forms, namely 24 hour R.O. and class R.O. Twenty-four hour R.O. involves the active participation of ward staff throughout the 24 hours in reorientating the patient for time, place and person on every occasion they interact with him. They use specially designed clocks, blackboards, signs, and posters placed strategically in the ward to facilitate their efforts. Class R.O. is comprised of daily half hour periods of intensive cognitive retraining for small groups run by a therapist. Recent research suggests that 24 hour R.O. not only improves cognitive functioning but also behaviour, while class R.O. only improves cognitive functioning. Twenty-four hour R.O. is also cheaper. If no treatable cause for this patient's confusion is found it would be well worthwhile placing him on a ward where R.O. is practised and it is likely that he will benefit up to the time when the progress of his illness, will make the therapy irrelevant.

Q7.
There has been a flourish of studies recently on the possible benefits of administering cholinergic substances to patients with memory disturbances, particularly those with Alzheimer's disease. There are sound a priori reasons to indicate that such substances should work. For example the administration of an anticholinergic such as hyoscine to healthy young adults results in a selective temporary memory deficit, similar to what may be found in elderly subjects. It has also been demonstrated that there is a deficiency of acetylcholine synthesis and of choline acetyltransferase activity in temporal lobe biopsy specimens from patients with Alzheimer's disease. However, administration of cholinergic substances to patients with Alzheimer's disease, has not resulted in very encouraging results, even though slight improvement in some has been reported within very narrow dosage ranges. It is unlikely that cholinergic sub-

stances, in our present state of knowledge, are indicated or would prove efficacious for this patient.

Course and management

The patient was admitted to a general hospital for investigations which were in general negative and no treatable cause for the confusion was found. Psychometric testing showed the patient to be 'functioning at a severely limited level in all areas of cognitive functioning, with a pattern of response strongly suggestive of generalised organic brain dysfunction'. The patient was transferred to a psychiatric hospital for further assessment. There was no improvement over a four month period. Consensus opinion viewed the patient as suffering with pre senile dementia, of undiagnosed type, but Pick's disease was suggested as a possibility. It was thought that on-going hospitalisation would be unavoidable.

Further reading

Christie J E, Shering A, Ferguson J, Glen A I M 1981 Physostigmine and arecoline: effects of intravenous infusions in Alzheimer presenile dementia. Brit J Psychiat 138: 46–50

Cutting J 1978 The relationship between Korsakoff's syndrome and 'alcoholic dementia'. Brit J Psychiat 132: 240–251

Enoch M D, Trethowan W H 1979 In: Uncommon psychiatric syndromes, 2nd edn, John Wright and Sons Ltd, Bristol, p 77–94

Granville Grossman K 1981 Hysterical symptoms in medicine. In: Readings in psychiatry, Hoechst Cotswald Press Ltd, Oxford

Kiloh L G 1975 Psychiatric disturbances of organic origin. Medicine (Second series) 10: 460–468

McGuire R J, Boyd W D 1981 Reality orientation and dementia: a controlled trial of two approaches. Brit J Psychiat 138: 10–14

CASE 51

A 56-year-old woman is brought to an emergency psychiatric clinic by her general practitioner. The patient is agitated, tearful and requests the doctor to, 'Please help me, admit me to hospital, I've lost my confidence, I won't get well any more, for God's sake get me well'. The general practitioner states that the patient has recently come onto his list, he doesn't know her very well and that she was taking phenelzine 15 mg and diazepam 5 mg six hourly up to two or three weeks ago. The patient is capable of giving a history with the support of her husband. The patient was adopted at about the age of three after both parents died accidently. She knows little of her natural parents but thinks they had no history of psychiatric illness. The adopting parents had two other older siblings, the father was a clerk in a county court and overall she got on well with the family. She was an average student at school and left at 16 without taking examinations. She worked in an office for a few years and subsequently for a period in the A.T.S. during the Second World War. Later she returned to office work and got married at the age of 28 to a local council administrator. There are four children of the marriage and all are well, and she claims that her marriage has been satisfying emotionally and sexually. She smokes and drinks moderately and describes herself as 'very sensitive, a great worrier, and at present very frightened and panicky'. She has no 'interests' outside the home setting. She was referred to psychiatric out-patients two years previously when she was told she was suffering from anxiety and was prescribed phenelzine and diazepam. Although she remained anxious the medication helped, but it was omitted when she was admitted to a general hospital two weeks previously for investigations of chest pains which were negative. The onset of symptoms was fairly quick, shortly after leaving hospital and coincided with the death of a favourite aunt. Over a period of a week she became increasingly tense and agitated, lost all confidence in herself, could not concentrate and became tearful. Her husband had to remain off work to comfort and reassure her, and she was afraid to go out even when accompanied by him. Her sleep is disturbed in that she has difficulty in getting off to sleep. She complains, 'I can feel my heart beating, I have butterflies in my tummy and feel weak in the legs'. She denies feeling depressed but says she is disgusted and angry with herself for feeling as she does and she does not entertain suicidal intent. On examination the patient is obviously anxious, tense and in a psychologically aroused state. Her pupils are moderately dilated, her pulse rate is 88 per minute and regular, her blood pressure is 140/90 and there is a slight increase in respiratory rate and a coarse tremor of her outstretched hands which are rather cold and moist.

Questions

1. What is the differential diagnosis?

2. Do you know of psychiatric conditions which may be drug induced?

3. If drugs are indicated for this patient's treatment, how would you rationalise your choice?

4. What theories on the central mechanism of action of benzodiazepines do you know of?

5. What do you know of the prevalence of psychiatric illness in general practice?

6. What are your views on the etiological significance of this patient's loss of both parents at the age of three, on her psychiatric state?

7. What are the indications for psychotherapy in the treatment of anxiety?

8. How would you manage this patient?

9. Comment briefly on the statement - 'The bulk of mental illness in any community never comes to the attention of psychiatrists'.

Answers

Q1.
The most likely diagnosis is an acute on chronic anxiety state. This is characterised by restlessness, agitation, apprehension and a high state of psychological arousal. She also has accompanying somatic signs such as palpitations, fast pulse, 'butterflies in the tummy', coarse tremor of the hands and cold moist palms. The admission to hospital for investigations and the death of a close relative may have been of importance in precipitating her present state. Also,

of course, she has a history of anxiety and is a sensitive anxious personality. It must also be kept in mind that the rather abrupt withdrawal of her long term medication especially the benzodiazepines exacerbated her condition and produced withdrawal effects, as she may have been dependent. Although the patient denies subjective depression, there is considerable overlap between symptoms of anxiety and depression (anxiety is present in over 80 per cent of patients suffering from a depressive illness), so there may be a depressive basis to her symptoms. Schizophrenia can be ushered in with acute anxiety, but there are no other symptoms supportive of this diagnosis and it would be uncommon for a schizophrenic illness to appear for the first time at the age of 56. The patient may be a vulnerable personality who is simply reacting negatively to stress. It is desirable to exclude such organic conditions as thyrotoxicosis, paroxysmal tachycardia and spontaneous hypoglycaemia. All these conditions are, of course, far less common than anxiety states. In thyrotoxicosis the tremor is fine, not coarse, the hands are warm not cold and clammy, the increased pulse rate will not slow during sleep and the patients always look far more anxious than they admit to. Paroxysmal tachycardia is characterised by a history of bouts of palpitations with a very fast heart rate, much faster than in anxiety states. An E.C.G. during a paroxysm will clarify the diagnosis. Spontaneous hypoglycaemia is characterised by relief of symptoms with taking food. Tumours of the adrenal medulla may give rise to symptoms suggestive of anxiety but the urine will contain large quantities of catecholamine metabolites.

Q2.

Indiscriminate unmonitored drug prescribing especially for patients on long term medication is most likely to lead to drug induced psychiatric conditions. Included in these conditions are depression, delirium, hypomania, paranoid and schizophrenic-like psychoses, hallucinatory states and pseudodementias. Depressive reactions to drugs vary from mild mood changes with loss of concentration and interest, to deep depression with nihilistic delusions and suicidal thoughts. The drugs most commonly incriminated in producing these effects are hypertensive drugs such as reserpine and methyldopa, major tranquillisers such as fluphenazine and flupenthixol, and analgesics - namely pentazocine and indomethacin. Miscellaneous drugs which may cause depression include corticosteriods, oral contraceptives and levodopa. Withdrawal from stimulants such as amphetamines and fenfluramine may be associated with depression.

Delirium ranging from apathy and perplexity to excitement and panic with visual hallucinations, may be drug induced especially in the elderly physically ill. Included among the offending drugs in the elderly are antidepressants, hypnotics, barbiturates, digoxin, hypotensives, phenothiazines and diuretics. The most commonly implicated drugs for all ages are phenothiazines, benzodiazepines, barbiturates and tricyclic antidepressants. Delirium may also be observed during withdrawal from alcohol, chlormethiazole, benzodiazepines and barbiturates.

Euphoric states ranging from mild euphoria to rarely frank hypomania may be induced by corticosteriods, A.C.T.H., opiates and pentazocine. Suppression of lactation in the puerperium by bromcriptine has produced mania. It is thought that the precipitation of mania by tricyclic or monoamine oxidase inhibitor antidepressants may reflect the presence of an underlying bipolar psychosis rather than an adverse drug reaction.

A large list of drugs have potential for producing paranoid or schizophrenic-like psychoses. Included are C.N.S. stimulants such as amphetamines and appetite suppressants, C.N.S. depressants such as alcohol and anticonvulsants, cardiovascular drugs such as digitalis and methyldopa, antiparkinsonion drugs such as levodopa and bromcriptine and, of course, hallucinatory drugs such as lysergide, mescaline, psilocybin and cannibis. Miscellaneous drugs and metals such as corticosteriods, A.C.T.H., lead and arsenic and vegetable poisons from mushrooms and derivatives of ergot are also incriminated.

Hallucinatory states may occur in isolation from other features of psychosis or delirium and can be induced by psychotropic drugs such as tricyclic antidepressants and benzodiazepines, by analgesics such as pentazocine and salicylates, and by cardiovascular drugs such as digitalis and beta blockers. The hallucinations are usually visual.

Pseudodementia is a word used to describe the condition of depression in the elderly, presenting with confusion. Some drugs, however, can produce a type of chronic delerious state in the elderly with many of the features of pseudodementia. The drugs most often culpable are major tranquillisers, barbiturates, tricyclic antidepressants, digoxin and antiparkinsonian drugs.

Apart from producing well recognised psychiatric syndromes, drugs may, of course, produce behavioural disorders distinct from these syndromes. For example violence and hypersexuality has resulted from combined levodopa-carbidopa therapy, lithium and neuroleptic drugs combined are reported to have induced sleep-walking and beta blockers and reserpine have been associated with nightmares.

Q3.

Many compounds apparently unrelated in their biochemical mechanism of action are clinically therapeutic in various forms of anxiety. In diagnostically undifferentiated anxiety (which might be an appropriate description for this woman's condition) benzodiazepines are certainly the most commonly used substances and may be most appropriate. From first interview it is not quite clear whether this woman suffers from associated sudden panic attacks with sweating, trembling, palpitations, and rapid breathing, as tricyclic antidepressants such as imipramine, or an M.A.O.I., are claimed to be effective in these states when benzodiazepines fail. As this woman also has some associated agoraphobia, an M.A.O.I. claimed to be effective in its treatment might be considered. In the treatment of anxiety states with pronounced somatic symptoms, a beta-adrenergic blocking drug such as propranolol may also be considered. A programme of supervised therapeutic trial and error of various anxiolytics singly and in combination may be the wisest strategem to follow, as there is no absolute clear cut rationale for a choice of drugs, which will consistently result in benefit to the individual patient.

Q4.

The central mechanism of action of benzodiazepines in the nervous system is still speculative to a large extent. Although several neurotransmitter substances have been postulated to be associated with their pharmacological action, the role of gama amino butyric acid (G.A.B.A.) has received most attention. Among the substances which have also been studied are glycerine, serotonin, cyclic A.M.P. and acetylcholine. It has been proposed that G.A.B.A. is the neurotransmitter which mediates presynaptic inhibition, and it is known that diazepam has a similar effect in the spinal cord. It has been proposed that diazepam may act by enhancing the action of G.A.B.A. neurones. Effects similar to those produced by diazepam have been produced by substances such as amino-oxyacetic acid and hydroxylamine which increase endogenous brain G.A.B.A. levels. Also G.A.B.A. has similar anticonvulsant, muscle relaxant and ataxic effects to diazepam. However, there is no evidence of an anti-anxiety role for G.A.B.A. Benzodiazepines have been described as mimicking the antianxiety, anticonvulsant and muscle relaxant effects of glycerine at its central nervous system sites. The glycerine receptor affinity of benzodiazepines, however, is inadequate to account for its anti-anxiety effect. Serotonin has also been implicated in the anti-anxiety mechanism of action of benzodiazepines. Substances which deplete serotonin from the nervous system were noticed to have anxyiolytic effects and in rats treated with these substances there was a blockade of chlordiazepoxide's activity. Results, however, are conflicting and the precise relationship between benzodiaze-pines and serotonin in the relief of anxiety is unknown. It has also been postulated that the anxiety reducing properties of benzodi-azepines such as diazepam and chlordiazoxide are mediated through inhibition of the enzyme which degrades cyclic A.M.P. namely cyclic A.M.P. phosphodiesterase. Many observers feel that this is not a very significant effect. It is probable that benzodiazepines undergo complex reactions with more than one neurotransmitter in effect-ing their many influences, and research in this exciting field is progressing.

Q5.
Although exact prevalence rates are difficult to ascertain it is thought that between a quarter to a third of all illness treated by general practitioners could be categorised as psychiatric. This does not imply that the general practitioner sees all the patients with psychiatric illness in his practice, nor does it give a clear cut indication of the size of the burden placed on the general practitioner by psychiatric patients. In some conditions where there is a loss of insight, or where there is marked agoraphobia the patient may not seek help. Also not every psychiatric problem is identified as such by a general practitioner, as the patient may present with somatic symptoma-tology of psychogenic origin. Commentators on psychiatric illness in general practice have divided the illnesses into major and minor. The major group is comprised of functional and organic psychoses, chronic alcoholism and severe subnormality. The minor group is comprised of neuroses in general and mild subnormality. Probably most of the psychiatric morbidity encountered by the general prac-titioner comes into the minor group. It has also been found that psychiatric patients make more demands on the general prac-titioner for general medical attention than non-psychiatric patients. They are also more likely to present members of the primary care team in the practice with associated family and social problems. It is difficult therefore to accurately assess the true prevalence of psychiatric illness in general practice or the burden carried by an individual practice. Also the wider availability of primary care

multdisciplinary teams in the future may change the pattern of contact and presentation.

Q6.

It is of course very difficult to state precisely in the individual case what psychological disadvantages, if any, an individual experiences due to the early loss by death of one or both parents. In general the effects of bereavement can be described for the child and the adult. Surprisingly there is little evidence that the death of a parent or parents in childhood directly produces adverse effects in later childhood or adolescence. At most there is only a slight increase in psychiatric disturbance and no relationship with childhood neurosis has been found. The psychological development of the child is of course influenced by many factors, environmental, educational and social which may in turn be influenced by the death of a parent. Parental death may therefore indirectly influence the child psychologically, but this influence may not always be adverse. It is thought by some that as parental death represents such a profound disturbance of family life more psychological ill effects in the child would be found if research techniques with more refined measurements were available. It is quite probable that in some cases childhood bereavement has 'sleeper' effects which only become apparent in adulthood, such as an increased susceptibility to depressive disorders, and to early divorce in men. It is quite possible that the psychological consequences of childhood bereavement may vary with the age of the child, and children in the two to three years old group may be most vulnerable. As this patient was in that age group at the time of her bereavement, it may have had an ill effect on her psychological development, but it is difficult to be conclusive.

Q7.

Anxiety states frequently have differential features which need different treatment methods. There is a place for psychotherapy alone or in combination with pharmacotherapy in the successful treatment of anxiety. Indeed there are many studies which demonstrate the superiority of combined psychotherapy and pharmacotherapy to either therapy used alone. Psychotherapy is thought to be indicated for treating the cognitive aspects of anxiety, that is the individual's interpretation of his somatic state. It is held that it is the individual's cognition which maintains the anxiety state. Although supportive psychotherapy and behaviour therapy are most commonly used there is little evidence to support the superiority of any one psychotherapeutic modality over another. A rational combination of combined treatment can be planned depending on the prominence of somatic and cognitive symptomatology. For example, when cognitive and somatic symptoms are high as in a panic state then pharmacotherapy comprised of antidepressants such as tricyclics or M.A.O.I. or beta blockers, combined with psychotherapy could be indicated. When cognitive symptoms are high and somatic symptoms are low as in generalised anxiety then psychotherapy would be most important and a benzodiazepine could be used in conjunction. When somatic symptoms are high but cognitive symptoms are low then a beta blocker may be of prime importance but the combination with psychotherapy would still be advisable.

Q8.
As this patient is so acutely anxious she should be admitted to hospital for observation. Admission to hospital and reassurance may have a beneficial effect and the exhibition of drugs may not be necessary. If her condition is due to abrupt withdrawal of drugs then it should gradually subside over a week or two. Full physical assessment will indicate if there is an organic basis to her symptoms. A sociopsychiatric report will indicate if there is an ongoing anxiety provoking factor in the patient's home or family life. Should the patient not improve over a period of time with hospitalisation and psychotherapy then it may be necessary to introduce pharmacotherapy. In the first instance a benzodiazepine such as diazepam could be prescribed starting with a low dosage such as 2 mg 6 hourly and if necessary increasing to 10 mg 6 hourly. It is probably preferable if possible to control her symptoms with one drug and avoid the introduction of a second. The combination of a benzodiazepine and an antidepressant such as phenelzine may be unavoidable. Supportive psychotherapy should continue concurrently and after the patient has been discharged she should be monitored frequently at outpatients. Manipulation of the patient's environment and attendance for a while at a day hospital may be indicated. The diagnosis should be reviewed if the patient failed to respond to the above measures.

Q9.
This statement is accurate. It has been estimated that 25 per cent of the population have significant psychiatric symptoms and less than 5 per cent can be identified as psychotic, or suffering from major mental illness. Psychiatrists tend mainly to come in contact

with psychotics. The remainder who suffer with mood disorders, psychosomatic symptoms, emotional distress and quite frequently severe depression will go to their general practitioner for treatment or get support from social workers, voluntary agencies or self help groups. Treating patients with minor psychiatric illnesses may take up about 1/3 of the general practitioner's time. It has been estimated that over 90 per cent of psychiatric finance is spent on hospital based services and psychiatrists spend 70 to 80 per cent of their time working within hospital settings. The inadequacy of community psychiatric care facilities has received much comment. There is a need to review the allocation of psychiatric finance and the traditional role of the hospital psychiatrist.

Course and management

The patient was admitted to hospital and was diagnosed as suffering from an acute on chronic anxiety state. She was treated with diazepam 5 mg 6 hourly after she failed over a period of two weeks to respond to supportive psychotherapy alone. She made a good response and was discharged on the same treatment to attend a day hospital once weekly.

Further reading

Clare A, Davies G 1979 Psychiatry in general practice. In: Hill. Murray, Thorley (eds) Essentials of postgraduate psychiatry, Academic Press, London, New York, p 567–598

Costa E, Greenjard P 1975 Mechanism of action of benzodiazepines. In: Advances in biochemical psychopharmacology 14, Raven Press Publishers, New York, p 1–28

Davidson K 1981 Toxic psychosis. Brit J Hosp Med 26(5): 530–537

Freedman A M, Dornbush R L, Shapiro B 1981 Anxiety: here today and here tomorrow. Comp Psychiat 22(1): 44–53

Greenwood J 1982 Community psychiatry in Edinburgh. Psychiatry in practice 22(1): 44–53

Rutter M 1972 Relationships between child and adult psychiatric disorders. Acta Psychiat Scand 48: 3–21

CASE 52

A 58-year-old man is returned to a psychiatric hospital by his 64-year-old brother. He left the hospital the previous day without informing the staff. His brother states he came to his house the previous evening and he took him in overnight and continues, 'but I cannot cope with him and his difficult behaviour'. The patient had been an inpatient in the hospital for about two weeks prior to leaving and had been referred by his brother's general practitioner, with a diagnosis of depression and subnormality. There is a history of numerous previous psychiatric admissions including admissions to subnormality and special hospitals dating back over a period of about 40 years. He also had many periods of imprisonment varying from three months to two and a half years, for crimes of petty theft and drunk, disorderly and aggressive behaviour. He always absconds from hospital. Reports from other hospitals describe him as suffering from subnormality, subnormality with a superimposed psychosis, or subnormal with a behaviour disorder and as a social problem. He was never a serious physical threat. The family and early history is obtained from his brother. The patient was the third of six siblings of working class parents and attended 'a school for backward children'. No other member of the family presented with a similar problem. He does not read or write. After leaving school at the age of 14 he adopted a type of vagrant life style and wandered about doing occasional labouring work at which he never persevered for more than a week or two. He never settled down or married. He has remained in good physical health, but is described in one report as exhibiting a coarse parkinsonian-like tremor which affects his hands, arms and head when he is under stress. At interview the patient shows little interest in the proceedings and appears intellectually incapable of giving a coherent account of himself. In appearance he looks more like a man of 70, than 58-years of age. There is no evidence of psychosis at present but one hospital report described him as 'hallucinated and paranoid'. He is restless and agitated rather than depressed and frequently asks, 'Can I come back to hospital?' Overall he gives the impression of poor intellectual endowment. During his previous hospitalisation physical investigations were negative and his Wechsler I.Q. assessment showed him to function at a verbal level of 61, a performance level of 63, and to have a full scale I.Q. of 60. During the course of his long psychiatric history he has been treated at different times with antidepressants, neuroleptics and E.C.T. At present he is receiving thioridazine 50 mg 6 hourly.

Questions

1. What is your formulation on this patient?

2. Does a patient described as a 'social problem' need the attention of a psychiatrist?

3. What is your concept of social psychiatry?

4. Comment on the statement — 'The development of community care will make the traditional large mental hospital redundant before the end of the century'.

5. In general, would it be more appropriate to describe as 'psychogeriatric', those patients aged 75 and upwards rather than as at present, those aged 65 and upwards?

6. Is it unavoidable that patients similar to this man will continue to present with a long history of numerous hospitalisations and imprisonments?

7. Would you comment on the statement — 'Mental hospital and prison populations are inversely related'?

8. Do you know of any criticism of the 1959 Mental Health Act for England and Wales?

9. Would you consider this patient fit to plead?

Answers

Q1.

This 58-year-old man could probably be best described as suffering from subcultural subnormality and presenting as a social problem. There is little evidence that he has ever been able to cope for long in the community since he left school in his teens and adopted a vagrant life style. There is a history of psychotic illness, but there is no evidence of this illness at present. He has a history of numerous psychiatric hospitalisations and imprisonments over a period of more than 40 years. His tendency to engage in petty theft may be indicative of his general social incompetence and inability to persevere at work, and is the main cause of his numerous imprisonments. It is most likely that the possibilities of success of any long term management and treatment programme have been severely compromised by his habit of absconding from hospital. His anti-social behaviour, non-compliance with treatment programmes in conjunction with his very poor intellectual endowment has probably made him unwelcome in many general psychiatric hospitals. Placement in a medium secure unit where he would have considerable freedom with an acceptable life style is probably indicated in the first instance. There would then be time to plan a long term management programme which might result in a more humane alternative life style. Institutional long stay care of some form will probably be unavoidable as he grows older.

Q2.

The term 'social problem' is commonly used in psychiatric practice to refer to individuals who come into contact with psychiatric services but present with problems apparently directly caused by or related to adverse social factors. In practice the term also implies that the social worker by alleviating the adverse social stress will largely solve the individual's problem and that there is little or no indication for psychiatric intervention. To accept such a limited view would not be in accord with the tenets of social psychiatry which is concerned with research into the social causes and consequences of psychiatric illness and with the application of social methods to its understanding and treatment. Depending on the individual details of the case, the attention of the psychiatrist and the social worker or of one or neither may be indicated. But the relationship between psychiatric illness and social factors in frequently complex and dynamic. The illness may be caused by or exacerbated by an adverse social environment or conversely the illness may result in the creation or exacerbation of adverse social factors. In general, it is advisable for a joint psychosocial approach to be made to the great majority of individuals who come into contact with psychiatric services labelled as 'social problems'. Such an approach will greatly help to elucidate if there is a relationship between the 'social problem' and psychiatric illness in the individual case.

Q3.

Social psychiatry is concerned with the study of the influence of social factors on the onset, duration and outcome of psychiatric conditions. It has focussed its attention on such questions as the distribution of suicide among the social classes and its relationship to family structure, the geographic distribution of psychiatric disorders within cities, and the links between psychiatric disorders and migration. The effect of the social atmosphere in institutions on their residents has also been studied. Although these epidemiological studies have been of great value, they cannot alone determine the direction of cause and effect, as they are natural rather than experimental studies. Social psychiatry has moved into the field of contrived experiment, with observation of the effect of manipulation of the environment on the individual.

Q4.

This statement is probably inaccurate. The run-down in the numbers of patients in the large mental hospital in the 1960s and early 1970's gave rise to a false sense of optimism in many observers. The enthusiasm to close the mental hospital and concentrate on treating patients in the community and in modern purpose built units in the setting of general hospitals, was both strong and infectious. The public image of the mental hospital was not good, they were considered as total institutions leading to chronicity and dependence in the patients, due to low standards of patient care and little rehabilitative effort. Reports of ill treatment of patients were not uncommon. Although the population of patients of most of these hospitals was reduced by $\frac{1}{3}$ to $\frac{1}{2}$ over a 10 year period, large numbers of 'hard core' patients still remained. This population was comprised primarily of two groups, namely a chronic long stay psychotic group and a psychogeriatric group, both presenting special difficulties for rehabilitation and discharge. Most of the psychotic group were so deteriorated socially that even if optimum residential community care were available, they would not succeed in remaining out of hospital. The psychogeriatric group needed continuous nursing and residential care which the local authorities could not provide. 'New chronic' patients continue to be admitted to the large mental hospitals and most now have a waiting list for psychogeriatric patients. Consensus opinion strongly favours the view that the large British mental hospital is likely to remain an essential part of the psychiatric service until at least the end of the century. Most of these hospitals have now been upgraded and modernised and are very active treatment and research centres, spearheading advances in rehabilitation and treatment.

Q5.

It is common practice in Britain to describe psychiatric patients aged 65 and upwards as psychogeriatric. Although 65 is the age when most people retire, get pensions, and are generally regarded as in

the old age group there are no clinically sound reasons for desig-
nating all psychiatric patients from this age upwards as psychogeriatric. It is a truism that the individual is unique in his physical and
mental strengths and weaknesses. There are many physically and
cognitively well preserved 75 to 85 year-old individuals treated for
depression both as outpatients and inpatients to whom it would be
a great injustice to place them in a psychogeriatric ward with cognitively impaired physically frail patients. Conversely it is not
uncommon to see patients in their 50s so deteriorated mentally and
physically that the adjective psychogeriatric would be appropriate.
The vast majority of individuals in the 65 to 74 years age group are
of course cognitively intact and far less likely than the 75 to 84 age
group to present with cognitive disturbance especially dementia. The
65 to 74 years age group will present largely with functional disorders and the 75 to 84 years age group with organic disorders
especially irreversible dementia. It could be argued that it would
be more fitting in general to describe as psychogeriatric patients aged
75 and upwards. The 65 to 74 years age group (60 per cent of the
elderly) would be absorbed into the general psychiatric fold, and
the psychogeriatric team could concentrate on using their limited
resources and specialist skills on those most in need. The percentage of old people in the 75 to 84 years old group is expected to increase
considerably over the next 20 years and make most demands on health
and social service facilities.

Q6.

It is likely at least for the immediate future that psychiatric patients
similar to this patient will follow a life style dominated by imprisonment and psychiatric hospitalisation. The facilities for treatment
and management of forensic psychiatric patients have for long been
inadequate. Judges occasionally comment that they have no alternative but to send an individual to prison when some other institution with an emphasis on psychiatric care would be more
appropriate, if such a facility were readily available. There is a
reluctance by psychiatrists to accept mentally abnormal offenders
especially those with a history of violence as they claim not to be
able to cope with them or retain them in hospital. With the introduction of new psychotropic drugs in the 1950s and 1960s and the
implementation of the 1959 Mental Health Act with its emphasis
on informal admission a new liberal attitude prevailed in the large
mental hospitals. The populations of the hospitals fell dramatically
and they boasted that they now had few or no locked wards. It is
now rather paradoxical that these advances in psychiatric practice

so beneficial in many ways, have resulted in the impotence of present day mental hospitals to contain and treat forensic psychiatric patients. The few special hospitals in the country are overcrowded and many patients who should be treated in semi-secure units if they were available in psychiatric hospitals are caught up in a revolving door between prison and community. When they are inadvertently admitted to their local psychiatric hospital they are likely to be re-referred or discharged when their forensic background is discovered. In an effort to rectify these shortcomings the Department of Health examined the problem and recommended that each Health Region in England and Wales should build a regional secure unit. There are now three or four such units. There have been considerable difficulties encountered in running these units, because their purpose has not been fully understood by psychiatrists. They are to provide assessment and formulate management plans for forensic patient, but not all forensic patients need admission to these units. Also they can only operate effectively if the hospitals in the regions they serve have medium secure units able to accept patients both from the community and from the secure unit. There would then be a turnover of patients and the unit could play a central role in training staff for forensic practice, provide advice and support for the medium secure units and be an impetus to research. Unless a sufficient number of medium secure units are set up in mental hospitals and these hospitals are willing to accept responsibility for forensic patients in their catchment areas then the purpose of the secure units will not be fully realised and patients similar to this patient are likely to continue to present with histories of numerous imprisonments and hospitalisations.

Q7.

This statement is not to be accepted literally nor indeed has it been established that prison populations rise in proportion to the fall in psychiatric hospital populations. Frequently this statement is used to emphasise that a high percentage of the prison population could be placed within psychiatric diagnostic categories and treated in hospital but the psychiatric service may be unwilling or has not the facilities, to treat them. The percentage of prisoners meriting a psychiatric diagnosis varies from 10 per cent to 90 per cent according to various estimates. In one survey in Britain on a representative sample of prisoners, 46 per cent were diagnosed as having a psychiatric disorder; 2 per cent were psychotic, 2 per cent were neurotic, 13 per cent were psychopathic, 11 per cent were alcoholic, less than 1 per cent were drug dependent and 14 per cent were subnormal or borderline subnormal, 1 per cent were epileptic and 2 per cent had other organic states. One American study regarded 52 per cent of a male prison population as suffering from a psychiatric condition other than sociopathy. Although hospital populations have decreased and prison populations increased in the last 30 years, the fall in one may not necessarily be associated with the rise in the other. Also it has not been clearly established that psychiatric patients in general have more innate criminal tendencies than the general population, and of course, imprisonment especially for long periods is conducive to the development of psychopathology. Nevertheless the concensus psychiatric opinion is that many individuals in prison would be more appropriately placed in psychiatric hospitals capable of retaining and treating them.

Q8.

The Mental Health Act (1959) (which is applicable only to England and Wales) was broadly based on the recommendations of a Royal Commission established to examine legal acts relating to mental disorder. This commission sat from 1954 to 1957. The objectives of the Act were to encourage informal admission, and where compulsory admission was necessary it was to be provided by recommendations of concurring medical practitioners without legal process or sanction and to provide safeguards to the rights of psychiatric patients. The act is generally regarded as a very important milestone in the development of a more humane approach in British psychiatric practice. It was formulated during a period when psychiatry was in a euphoric phase. New treatments, particularly more effective drug treatments for the major psychoses were controlling the more unpleasant aspects of these illnesses and the population of the large mental hospital was falling. Criticism of the Act has centred mainly on the misuse of compulsory powers and the inadequacy of safeguards. In 1975 a committee was established to review the Act and a white paper was published in 1978. Disquiet has been expressed by many observers especially by the National Association of Mental Health (MIND). The main criticisms are as follows: Informal admission is open to abuse as the patient may not be fully informed or appreciate the consequences of his admission and an unprotesting patient may be regarded as consenting. The Act lacks precision in defining mental disorder, and many forms of eccentric or unusual behaviour could come within the definition and hence the Act is open to abuse. Psychiatric diagnosis tends to be unreliable and and it is relatively easy to find two doctors prepared to make recommendations which may be inconsistent with the consensus medical view. A general practitioner or a social worker is likely to comply with the judgements and directions of a consultant psychiatrist when compulsory admission is considered. Section 29 of the Act which empowers one doctor to compulsorily admit a patient is open to misuse. The doctor completing the order may have little experience in psychiatry, and although the compulsory duration of hospitalisation is only 72 hours, the act of compulsory admission itself may be more psychologically traumatic than any subsequent duration of stay. Section 136 of the Act which enables a police officer to detain and take to a place of safety a person in a public place who appears to be suffering from a mental disorder has been criticised because the police officer is not competent to judge if a person is suffering from mental disorder and also the place of safety could mean a police cell within the definition. Section 25 of the Act permits a person to be compulsorily detained in hospital for 28 days observation. During this period, the courts will not hear a plea for habeas corpus and the patient has no rights to apply to a mental health tribunal. In practice patients are commonly treated against their will during this period of observation. A patient can be compulsorily detained for a year under provision of Section 26 of the Act. This period is regarded as too long and at variance with current advances in treatment. Mental Health Review Tribunals also established under the Act to ensure that compulsory patients were not detained unnecessarily, have also been criticised. It is thought that many patients do not apply to these tribunals, not because they accept their detention, but because they do not fully understand their rights and feel incompetent to cope with the procedure. Tribunals only have the power to discharge or leave in hospital, and it has been suggested that they should have further options such as the power to discharge the patient into a less restrictive setting such as a hostel or special home. It is now most probable that many of these criticisms will be met in the near future by new legislation. Proposals in the Mental Health (Amendment) Bill published in November 1981 would considerably strengthen patients' rights.

Q9.

This patient is probably not fit to plead. In assessing whether an individual is fit to plead it is the mental state at the present time and not the mental state at the time of the crime that is assessed. The psychiatrist must ascertain if the accused understands the following:

    (a) the nature and possible consequences of the charge
    (b) the difference between a plea of guilty and not guilty

(c) and is able to instruct his legal representatives
(d) challenge a juror
(e) follow the evidence in court.

If he is incapable of doing all of these things he should be considered under disability and unfit to plead. The present legistralation has been criticised because there is a danger than an individual may be regarded as a 'criminal lunatic' because of his unfitness to plead. Should the patient recover and and be fit to plead he may have to return to court and if found guilty may be compulsorily detained after already having spent a period of compulsory detention in hospital.

Course and Management

The patient was admitted to hospital informally. While plans were being formulated for long stay placement and management, the patient again left the hospital without informing staff and did not return to his brother's residence.

Further reading

Bewley T H, Bland M, Mechen D, Walch E 1981 New chronic patients. Brit Med J 283: 1161–1164

Gostin L O 1978 The Mental Health Act 1959. Is it fair? MIND (National association for mental health) special report

Gunn J 1977 Criminal behaviour and mental disorder. Brit J Psychiat 130: 317–329

Hemsi L 1980 Psychgeriatric care in the community. Health Trends 12: 25–29

Leff J 1978 Reading about social psychiatry. Brit J Psychiat 132: 516–517

Lloyd G G 1979 Social and transcultural psychiatry. In: Hill, Murray, Thorley (eds) Essentials of postgraduate psychiatry, Academic Press, London, New York, p 505–526

MIND 1981 New mental health bill welcomed by MIND. Mindout 55: 3

Swan M 1981 Fitness to plead. Brit J Hosp Med 25 (5): 503–509

CASE 53

A 39-year-old man is referred from casualty to a psychiatric hospital, because he informed the casualty officer that he was depressed and suicidal. He was treated in casualty for a laceration to his hand, received when he was assaulted while drinking in a club. Both parents are alive, but separated since the patient was eight years old, the patient is the second of three siblings. There is no psychiatric history in the family background. He had a reasonably happy childhood, was reared by his mother and visited regularly by his father with whom he got on well. The father was a clerk in the civil service. The patient was a reasonably good student, had many friends at school and did one 'A' and three 'O' levels. He entered university to study English and history but left after one year and got a job as a clerk. At the age of 27 he was admitted to hospital for the treatment of depression. He received E.C.T. and antidepressants, and appeared to make a good recovery but lost his job due to absenteeism. He had three more admissions to hospital between the ages of 27 and 31 for depression and suicidal attempts by overdosing with drugs. His most recent admission was one year previously when he presented in outpatients, intoxicated with alcohol, and stated that he felt suicidal. He is contentedly homosexual and is unmarried, and has not had a regular boy friend for two to three years, he smokes heavily and is inclined to drink heavily at week-ends, he also smokes hashish. He is well physically and describes himself as nervous, sensitive, interested in literature and the arts, and sociable with a small number of friends. At times he feels persecuted by society in general and he denies ever having been involved with the law or being in prison. He lives on social security as he finds it difficult to get a job. On examination he is well preserved, speaks well, spontaneously and to the point. He has a good vocabulary, uses many psychiatric phrases which he has probably learned during the course of his psychiatric history. There is no evidence of depression apart from unhappiness and sadness related to his poor life situation. He denies suicidal intent, there are no perceptual or cognitive disorders evident and he appears to be functioning at a good intellectual level.

Questions

1. What is your formulation on this patient?

2. Have you heard of any characteristics of adolescents who take overdoses?

3. What do you know of the etiology of personality disorder?

4. Very briefly criticise the concept of 'the neuroses'.

5. Comment briefly on the statement 'psychiatrists tend to diagnose personality disorder or psychopathy in patients whom they dislike or are unsuccessful in treating'.

6. How would you manage this patient?

7. What are the indications and limitations of group psychotherapy?

8. What do you know of cognitive therapy for the treatment of depression?

9. Comment briefly on the statement 'personal psychoanalysis is necessary for the training of a psychiatrist'.

Answers

Q1
A 39-year-old, unmarried, unemployed, homosexual man, with a long history of drug overdoses and psychiatric hospitalisations, is referred to a psychiatric hospital from a casualty department. He was treated for a lacerated hand sustained from an assault in a club. On arrival in hospital, he is found not to have overt psychiatric symptomatology, apart from dissatisfaction, sadness and loneliness related to an unhappy life situation, but in casualty he confessed to feeling depressed and suicidal. The most likely diagnosis at first interview is that he is suffering from a personality disorder, and the outlook in the short and medium term is not good.

Q2.
There is evidence to suggest that the epidemic of deliberate self-poisoning has peaked, however, the incidence among young people particularly in their early teens continues to rise. Studies have shown that the female to male ratio may be as high as 9 to 1. The great excess of females, is thought to be due to the earlier onset of adulthood with its sexual and relationship problems for females, and boys regard overdosing as culturally unacceptable. They may find an outlet for their distress in aggressive or violent behaviour. Young people frequently have a precipitant such as a row with parents or with a

boy friend. There is no evidence at present that the increase in adolescent self-poisoning is closely related to the increase in alcohol consumption among adolescents in general. There is also a high prevalence of recent general hospital admission and current physical illnesses among adolescent self-poisoners, and this partly explains the increased frequency of visits to the general practitioner prior to the overdose. During these visits, however, the young person does not discuss personal or psychiatric problems with the general practitioner. Referral for psychiatric hospitalisation after emergency treatment does not appear in general indicated for this group. Changes in prescribing habits will not reduce the frequency of self-poisoning, as in contrast to older groups who take tranquillisers, antidepressants and opiate analgesics, these adolescents take paracetamol or aspirin, which are readily purchased. They also have a much poorer relationship with parents than adolescents in general. Their problems tend to be transient but 14 per cent may be referred for further treatment of self-poisoning within a year.

Q3.

The etiology of personality disorder is ill understood. Genetic, biological, social and psychological factors all influence personality development and a disorder in any of these factors will adversely influence integrated personality growth. Twin studies have fairly well established that certain personality traits and intelligence are more likely to be concordant for MZ twins than for DZ twins. It is probably reasonable to conclude that adverse personality traits may to some degree be genetically determined. Animal experiments suggest that personality development and sexual orientation can be influenced during the intrauterine and neonatal period by drugs and hormones and of course by brain damage. This research is relevant to human personality development. Low birth weight children and those who suffer cerebral trauma during birth, even without neurological signs, may exhibit personality problems during the first decade of life. Separation from parents especially the mother in the early years of life may be very deleterious. Social and psychological factors thought to adversely influence personality development in children include a poor parental marital relationship or marital breakdown, lack of affection, encouragement and support from parents or teachers. Poor example from parents who may themselves have personality disorders, such as the exhibition of unwarranted aggressive or violent behaviour, will stimulate the child to model his behaviour pattern on a similar line. The plasticity of the developing personality responds to observed behaviour in parents, teachers and peers as in a learning situation. Although a degree of concretisation in personality development occurs in middle age, development is still discernible into late life and personality disorders may ameliorate over a period of time.

Q4.

Considerable discussion exists on the precise meaning of the term 'the neuroses'. The World Health Organisation definition lays stress on factors such as no demonstrable organic basis, retention of insight and contact with reality. The psychoses in contrast may have an organic basis, insight is lost and contact with reality may be tenuous. The presence of neurosis will be manifest by hysterical obsessional, compulsive, phobic or anxiety symptoms. In the eighteenth century the concept implied a disease of the nervous system and Freud and the analytic movement introduced the psychogenic aspect with fixation at the oral or anal level of psychological development as of etiological importance. The behavioural school have stressed the maladaptive and learning aspects in causation. That there are many views on definition, causation and treatment is indicative of how poorly the whole concept of 'the neuroses' is understood. What is the relationship to personality disorder, to other psychiatric illnesses, how justifiable and valid is the subdivision into neurotic types? The answers to these questions are far from complete. Reliability of diagnosis for 'the neuroses' has been found to be substantially lower than for psychoses or organic psychiatric illnesses, and as to the type of 'neurosis' present, reliability falls still further. The concept of 'neuroses' frequently gives little valid indication of prognostic and therapeutic implications because of variability of course. It has been claimed that any diagnosis which fails to embody strong prognostic and therapeutic implications is of little value. It has been suggested that a multi-dimensional approach to 'the neuroses', where, in the individual patient, the strength and weaknesses of his personality, the magnitude of stresses he is subjected to, the pattern of his responses, and the treatment programme are all studied, would be more meaningful and fruitful. The term has also been criticised as instilling a degree of therapeutic nihilism in doctors who may be inclined to believe that the main onus for improvement lies with the patient. However, although there are many shortcomings in the concept of 'the neuroses' the adjective 'neurotic' is very meaningful for the practising psychiatrist.

Q5.

The great reward in medicine is to see patients improve as a result of therapeutic endeavour and express gratitude to their doctor. In treating a patient with a personality disorder or with psychopathy, the psychiatrist may only see a minimal improvement after long delay or no improvement. During treatment the patient may not comply with the treatment regime, be very time consuming, make unreasonable demands, and be verbally or physically aggressive to the doctor. The temptation to describe the patient as incorrigible and relieve oneself of clinical responsibility may be great. In general, most psychiatrists resist this temptation, a minority may not.

Q6.

This patient should not be admitted to hospital as he probably is not now suicidal. There is no indication for psychotropic medication, but he should be seen in the near future at psychiatric outpatients. Some form of psychotherapy such as group therapy may be appropriate, and referral to an employment agency which specialises in obtaining employment for psychiatric patients may be indicated. It is quite possible that as one gets a greater knowledge of this patient at outpatient attendances, other treatment options such as more formal psychotherapy may be feasible.

Q7.

Group psychotherapy may be indicated for a wide variety of psychiatric conditions including neuroses, psychoses and personality disorders. Group therapy encompasses a variety of treatment approaches. Treatment goals may include overcoming social isolation, training in social skills, modifying maladaptive symptoms and encouraging reality-orientated behaviour. Treatment techniques also vary widely, and may include non verbal exercises, psychodrama and related experimental techniques, didactic sessions and education on symptoms and their precipitants. Psychoanalytical group therapy is of course common in the United States of America and this may take place conjointly with personal analysis. Ideally the group will be comprised of eight patients, all over the acute stage of their illnesses, the majority will suffer from neurosis or personality disorder, frequently with related social interaction problems. One or two quiescent psychotic patients may also be present. The limitations to present day group psychotherapy are many. Although there are many anecdotal claims for success, there is little evidence that a systematic body of knowledge is emerging in this field. The therapists are frequently poorly trained para medicals. Members of the group may run the risk of being pressurised and coerced into submission and respond with pseudochange which does not outlive the groups duration. The emphasis on insight into psychogenic conflicts is inappropriate in psychoanalytical groups, because of the short term duration of the therapy. Many of these limitations can be overcome by a well trained therapist skilled in selecting both the members of the group and an appropriate treatment technique.

Q8.
Cognitive therapy is a relatively new psychological treatment for several minor psychiatric disorders and depression. The outcome of studies in the United States of America and the United Kingdom are favourable. The aim of treatment in depression is to influence benignly the associated negative thoughts. To achieve this objective the patient is directed to keep a written record of all 'negative automatic thoughts' and of the events conducive to them. Over a a period of about 20 sessions the patient discusses with the therapist the thoughts which occurred since the last interview. The patient will be encouraged to substitute more realistic thoughts and beliefs and to plan his free time so that he will attain morale boosting or pleasurable achievements. The treatment is not based solely on encouragement and counter argument but also on the use of several therapeutic techniques in a highly structured form. It is claimed that cognitive therapy over a period of about 20 treatment sessions is as effective as the use of tricyclic drugs, while of course being free of side effects, and that outcome after 12 months is better. The therapy is time consuming, each session requiring on average 50 minutes, and training is needed in its mastery. The temptation for overburdened psychiatrists to quickly prescribe an antidepressant will remain strong.

Q9.
Personal psychoanalysis is not necessary for the training of a psychiatrist. Different patients demand different therapeutic approaches, and although it is desirable for the therapist to have a wide range of skills, none should be overvalued or exclusive of others. Many approaches help trainees to understand and empathise with patients, such as direct instruction, modelling, roleplay, and observed practice with immediate feedback using audio visual equipment. Few if any psychotherapists would argue that personal psychoanalysis is necessary in training. They would stress its value in helping the therapist to understand the functioning of his own mind, to avoid over or under involvement with patients and therapeutically damaging reactions to feelings provoked by them.

Course and management

After consultation it was decided to admit the patient informally to hospital for a short period of observation. Over a period of one week it was noted that he showed no evidence of depression and he was considered not to be suicidal. The patient was desirous of leaving and was discharged after eight days. Psychotropic medication was not prescribed and arrangements were made for further follow up at outpatients where other treatment options could be considered.

Further reading

Cox J, Marks M, Marteau L, Steiner J 1982 Personal psychotherapy in the training of a psychiatrist. Bull Roy Coll Psychiat 6 (3): 38–42

Goldberg D 1982 Cognitive therapy for depression. Brit Med J 284: 143–144

Hawton K, O'Grady J, Osborn M, Cole D 1982 Adolescents who take overdoses: their characterisics, problems and contacts with helping agencies. Brit J Psychiat 140: 118–123

Martin J M 1982 Genotype — environment interaction in antisocial behaviour. Psych Med 12(2): 235–239

Pallis D J, Barraclough B M, Levy A B, Jenkins J S, Sainsbury P 1982 Estimating suicide risk among attempted suicides. The development of new clinical scales. Brit J Psychiat 141: 37–44

Pollitt J 1982 Major common symptoms in psychiatry - sadness. Brit J Hosp Med 27(2): 117–120

CASE 54

A 47-year-old man is referred from a psychiatric emergency clinic for admission to hospital. He is described as 'A chronic alcoholic with depression and suicidal ideas'. Both parents are dead, he is the third of four siblings one of whom suffered with depression. There is no history of alcoholism in the family background, and he got on well with both parents. The father worked as a technical engineer. The patient was reasonably bright at school and left at the age of 16. He was apprenticed to the catering trade, and has worked as a caterer cum waiter ever since, but has been unemployed for the preceding two years. He married at 22 and has two children. His wife has been very supportive over many years, although subjected to frequent verbal abuse and infrequent violence. She accompanied him to outpatients and helped in providing a coherent history. He agreed to seek help because his wife threatened to leave him if he did not. He is described as rather tense and anxious and alcohol relieves his tension, he has few friends apart from 'old cronies' he meets in the pub and has few outside interests. He smokes heavily. He started drinking heavily about 20 years ago and has had three admissions to psychiatric hospitals with alcohol related problems, the first was 15 years previously, another about 12 years ago and the most recent was two years ago. He had periods of abstinence extending up to two years, but he invariably resumes drinking. His general physical health is good and there is no clinically apparent alcohol related physical damage. During the preceding 10 months he has drunk heavily, and claims to drink 'up to 20 pints a day when I can afford it'. His wife states that 'it is an exaggeration' and that he does not or cannot drink as heavily as previously. His sleep and appetite are poor, and he says he is depressed and states 'I wish to sleep and never wake up again'. He expresses general dissatisfaction with his life style and with his inability to get and hold down a job and he relates all his misfortunes to his problem with alcohol. On assessment he smells strongly of alcohol, there is no cognitive impairment or psychotic features evident. He appears miserable and tearful, rather than clinically depressed, and although he expresses a wish to die, there is no evidence of active suicidal ideation or behaviour. He admits to having a 'drinking problem' and says he realises he needs help and requests admission to hospital. Routine physical examination is negative, but he is probably overweight.

Questions

1. What is your formulation on this patient?

2. Do you know of psychological theories on the causation of alcoholism?

3. Is there no alternative to total abstinence from alcohol for this patient?

4. What do you know of the inheritance of alcoholism?

5. How do female alcoholics differ from male alcoholics?

6. Has hypnosis a role in the treatment of this patient?

7. What are the psychiatric applications of hypnosis?

Answers

Q1.

This 47-year-old man, who presented as a psychiatric emergency is suffering from chronic alcohol addiction of about 20 years duration. He is probably physically and psychologically dependent and although he appears to have insight he may be lacking motivation as he sought help only under pressure from his wife. His occupation as a waiter cum caterer may have been of importance in the causation of his problem and he is miserable rather than depressed. Although there is no clinical evidence of related organic damage and he has the support of his family, the prognosis is poor, because of poor motivation and probable underlying personality defects. He should be admitted for consideration of treatment options.

Q2.

There are numerous psychological theories on the causation of alcoholism. Many of them are considered far too allembracing and general and could be relevant to many personality and psychiatric problems. Some analysts relate alcohol addiction to unresolved parental relationships in early life which result in general dependence in adult life and this dependence is seen in many alcoholics. There is poor personality development, the immediate pleasure is grasped and the long term gain ignored, and this is how the individual deals with present anxiety. Behaviourists consider alcoholism as a form of maladaptive learning, which is treatable symptomatically by retraining. Classical conditioning theory proposes that one may be conditioned to the sight, smell and sound of drinking occasions as pleasurable in themselves when associated with pleasant alcohol induced feelings. Various personality characteristics have also been associated with alcoholism. These include individuals described as having identity problems, latent homosexuality or of being analytically orally fixated. There is, however, no established evidence of an alcoholic personality type although personality disturbance is frequently noted.

Q3.

Up to recent years, it has been customary to advise alcoholic patients to abstain totally from alcohol. There is considerable interest now in teaching some patients 'controlled' drinking by giving painful stimuli when they drink too quickly or take big mouthfuls in a simulated 'pub' setting. Total abstinence as the criterion of success has been criticised as too simplistic, and of course some abstinent alcoholics may be more disturbed than those taking alcohol. It is also incorrect to state that one drink will inevitably precipitate physiological craving and continuous drinking, and some patients may be tempted after one drink to make such a statement self-fulfilling. Patients treated by behavioural controlled drinking methods have done as well as patients treated by abstinent methods. Each case will have to be judged individually and there may be different forms of alcoholism needing different approaches. This patient's addiction is chronic and as he normally works in an occupation where he is exposed to alcohol, total abstinence may be indicated.

Q4.

Although alcoholism has been noted to be familial, this cannot be explained by hereditary or genetic factors alone as environment is also important. There are also large group differences in the prevalence of alcoholism due to social, cultural and racial influences, with variations from one historical era to another, from social class to social class and from country to country. It is safe to conclude that susceptibility to alcoholism is not entirely genetic, although well designed studies of adopted half siblings and twins do implicate genetic factors. Another difficulty in elucidating the precise role of hereditary factors is presented by the heterogeneity of alcoholism and alcohol related problems, in which nature, nurture, culture and race may have differing quantative influences. For example, two types of alcoholism have been described in the United States of America for which it is claimed there are distinct genetic and environmental causes and which differ in their association with criminality, severity of alcohol abuse and the frequency of expression in biological mothers. Further research on the constitutional pre-disposition to alcoholism must focus on more clearly defined sub-groups of alcoholics. The discrepancy in research findings may be explained by failure to do this.

Q5.

Female alcoholics are reported as differing considerably from their male counterparts. They are more likely to have a parent, spouse, or sibling with alcoholism and experienced more deprivation as children through divorce, desertion or death. Women tend to develop problems with alcohol at a later age than men, and to be admitted to psychiatric hospitals more frequently and have more broken marriages, and attempt suicide more frequently. They are described as having a shorter more 'telescoped' developmental period between early problem drinking and late stage symptoms. Women alcoholics are more likely to remain hidden by their families, and drink alone in the privacy of their home. The female alcoholic is more likely to have affective disorder while the male is likely to be sociopathic. Women are also reported as exhibiting more clear cut associated psychological stress factors. The weekly consumption of alcohol is probably less for women. Alcoholism among women would appear to be an increasing problem with the male to female ratio changing over 25 years from 7 to 1, to 4 to 1. Some commentators believe this reflects the greater availability of treatment facilites in recent years, others that it is due to the greater availability of alcohol in supermarkets and the changed life style of many women.

Q6.

In general, hypnosis in isolation has no role in the treatment of alcoholism. It has been used, however, in the treatment of the addictions (nicotinism, alcoholism and drugs) to achieve aversion in imagery, in conjunction with other forms of treatment and some success is claimed. As well as the addiction problem the alcoholic also frequently has related social, physical and psychiatric complications and may need a broad approach in treatment.

Q7.

Patients suffering from neurotic illness benefit most from hypnotherapy, and it may be used in conjunction with other forms of treatment. The patient may also eventually be taught autohypnosis or self hypnosis so that his reliance on the therapist will decline. Care must be exercised that an underlying untreated organic condition is not masked or that severe underlying depression responsive to other forms of treatment is recognised. Hypnosis has a place in the treatment of anxiety states, insomnia, psychosomatic illnesses, psychosexual problems (impotence, vaginismus, frigidity) hysterical conversion neuroses, phobic and obsessional compulsive states. The experienced therapist will know which technique to apply and how best to integrate it into a treatment programme.

Course and management

The patient was admitted to hospital but requested his discharge five days later when he was reconciled with his wife. It was arranged for him to be seen at outpatients by a psychiatrist in charge of an alcoholic unit and the patient agreed to keep this appointment on leaving hospital, but subsequently failed to do so. Further approaches by community staff were rebuffed.

Further reading

Cloninger R C, Bohman M, Sigvordrson S 1981 Inheritance of alcohol abuse. Arch Gen Psychiat 38(8): 861–867

Greenblatt M, Schuckit M A 1976 How women alcoholics differ from men alcoholics. In: Alcohol problems in women and children, Grune and Stratton, New York, p 73–74

Murray R M, Gurling H M D 1982 Alcoholism. Polygenic influence on a multifactorial disorder. Brit J Hosp Med 27(4): 328–334

Waxman D 1980 Clinical aspects of hypnosis in psychiatry. Brit J Hosp Med 23(5): 456–463

CASE 55

A man aged 37 has been admitted to several psychiatric hospitals within a period of a few years giving generally the same surname but a series of different first names. On each occasion he describes a similar story, claiming the recent death of one or both of his parents in a road traffic or other accident which has left him feeling depressed and suicidal; sometimes he has taken an overdose of drugs or cut his wrists. He says he can see and hear the deceased and is unable to accept the loss. He states that his sleep and appetite have been poor and he has generally been neglecting himself. He denies any previous psychiatric history but admits to homosexuality and sometimes describes recent difficulties in an apparently stable relationship. He claims to be a university graduate and to be working as a nurse or for a university. His mental state appears at first to be consistent with his story of bereavement and he spends much time on his bed and weeps freely at any reference to death, accidents etc. At times, however, he is observed to be apparently enjoying himself and mixing easily with other patients. His dramatic story and behaviour soon give rise to suspicion and investigation of his claims quickly reveals most to be untrue. Confrontation over the falsity of his statements does not, however, seem to upset him particularly and he usually leaves hospital soon afterwards.

Questions

1. Into what diagnostic category would you place this patient?

2. Who was Munchausen? Is there an alternative name for this condition?

3. With what sort of complaints do these patients usually present?

4. What etiological factors have been described in the Munchausen syndrome?

5. In what other conditions may pseudologia phantastica occur?

6. How should patients with this condition be managed?

7. Which psychiatric conditions may present in an acutely disturbed manner on general hospital wards?

Answers

Q1.
It is quite clear that this man repeatedly engineers his admission to psychiatric hospitals and units by fabricating a grief reaction. In this respect there is a close resemblance to patients who present with fictitious physical symptoms in order to gain admission, investigation and often treatment in general hospitals — a condition which was first given the name of Munchausen syndrome by Richard Asher, a general physician who worked in an 'observation ward' admitting psychiatric emergencies. Apart from the presence of mental rather than physical symptoms this patient's condition would appear to warrant the same diagnosis; i.e. a psychiatric Munchausen syndrome.

Q2.
Asher named this condition after Baron Munchausen who is said to have lived from 1720 to 1797 and to have served in the Russian army against the Turks. The Baron was supposed to have been in the habit of grossly exaggerating his exploits and these were published in an English version by a German, Rudolph Erich Raspe, in 1785 as 'Baron Munchausen, Narratives of his Marvellous Travels'. The choice of eponym has, however, been criticised on literary and clinical grounds since, firstly, the Baron himself did not actually feign illness (though like the patients he did travel widely) and secondly, the name tends to trivialise the condition. Other authors have suggested equally colourful names but Barker's 'hospital addiction' is less open to such criticisms.

Q3.
The usual Munchausen patient presents with physical symptoms in almost any part of the body. As with genuine organic disease, pain is the commonest complaint (often abdominal — named 'laparotomophilia migrans' by Asher!) and like any subjective symptom is impossible to disprove especially as it may be backed up with evidence of blood in vomit, sputum, urine etc. which patients may go to extraordinary lengths to achieve (Asher's 'haemorrhagica histrionica'). Neurological symptoms comprise another common presentation ('neurologica diabolica' of Asher) including headache, faints and fits. Not uncommonly there is some genuine condition such as an established cardiac arrhythmia or evidence of an old cardiac infarct with which the patient is able to bolster up

his complaints. Not only are the presenting symptoms very variable but they may differ in the same patient on different occasions.

The present patient differs, of course, in certain respects from the classical Munchausen patient in that he presents with a picture of a psychological rather than physical illness and so does not invite physical investigations and possible surgery.

Q4.

The most obvious feature of the condition is the desire to be considered ill and to be admitted to hospital often including the wish to undergo surgery. It has been pointed out that the motivation for this behaviour, abnormal though it is, probably arises from the same satisfactions — care, attention etc. — that are a normal accompaniment of illness and the 'sick role'. It is, however, exaggerated in the Munchausen patient and forms part of a more general pattern of psychopathy with, commonly a history of criminal behaviour, of a wandering and vagrant way of life and a tendency to colourful lying or pseudologia phantastica — a picture certainly shown by the present patient.

Q5.

The distinction between 'fantastic' lying and more common and less obvious distortions of the truth is clearly a matter of degree as is the extent of conscious awareness on the part of the individual. The term pseudologia phantastica should, perhaps, be reserved for the long standing or 'constitutional' tendency associated with psychopathy but similar dramatic fabrications may be expressed by patients with organic disease, especially G.P.I. Of course, in such cases there is complete lack of insight into their falsity and they are really elaborations of the patient's delusions. In the Munchausen syndrome it is often assumed that the patient is malingering and fully aware of his behaviour but it may well be that many are quite convinced of the reality of their complaints — at least at the time.

Q6.

A major difficulty in attempting to help these patients is their usual practice of discharging themselves as soon as their condition is recognised by the hospital staff. In fact their referral to a psychiatrist is uncommon and this is, perhaps, understandable in view of the failure so far of psychiatric treatment to effect any improvement even if contact with the patient can be maintained. Prolonged detention in a psychiatric hospital has, however, been recommended to prevent the self-destructive behaviour of some patients.

Q7.

Most psychiatric conditions can present in an acutely disturbed manner on a general ward. Disturbed behaviour may take many forms such as aggressive or violent behaviour towards staff or other patients, threats or attempts at suicide, or making excessive demands, or delirious states due to various causes or generalised over activity due to manic or schizophrenic states. Conditions commonly encountered are alcohol related withdrawal states, hypomanic and paranoid psychoses, acute and chronic schizophrenia, personality disordered patients especially those with drug related problems, patients in hysterical states and rarely a Munchausen Syndrome.

Course and management

The same treatment difficulties as those just described apply to the present patient with 'psychiatric' Munchausen syndrome. Despite confrontation he continues to be untruthful, declines any help that is offered, and usually discharges himself. When a community psychiatric nurse has been sent to visit him at home the address he has given on admission proves not to exist and his supposed general practitioner denies any knowledge of him. It is likely, therefore, that his pattern of frequent psychiatric admissions will continue.

Further reading

Asher R 1951 Munchausen's syndrome. Lancet 1: 339

Barker J C 1962 The syndrome of hospital addiction (Munchausen syndrome). J Ment Sci 108: 167

Blackwell B 1968 In: Silverstone J, Barraclough B (eds) Contemporary psychiatry, Headly Bros Ltd

Enoch MD, Trethowan W H 1979 The Munchausen syndrome and some related disorders. In: Uncommon psychiatric symptoms, John Wright and Sons Ltd, Bristol

Pfeffer J M 1981 Management of the acutely disturbed patient on the general ward. Brit J Hosp Med 26(1): 73–80

CASE 56

A 24-year-old married woman of Mauritian origin is transferred from a maternity ward to a psychiatric unit because of disturbed behaviour six days after the delivery of her first child. Her father is aged 55 and a shopkeeper in Mauritius. Her mother died at the age of 35 when the patient was four years old, possibly of heart disease. She has five brothers and three sisters. One of the brothers has epilepsy and one sister had a puerperal psychosis after her baby died soon after birth. The patient was brought up by foster parents after her mother's death until she was 15 years old. She attended school until the age of 11 years and then worked in shops and a factory before coming to England 16 months ago to marry her husband whom she had met in Mauritius and who had been in this country for five years. She denies any previous history of physical or psychiatric illness and is described by her husband as being a friendly, cheerful and sociable young woman. On admission she shows poor attention and concentration and looks somewhat bewildered, appearing not to know where she is and asking who people are despite being told repeatedly. She expresses the belief that some harm will befall her but it is sometimes difficult to follow the train of her thought because of apparent inexplicable connections between one thought and the next. Her affect appears at times to be inappropriate to her situation and thought content but at other times she seems to be depressed and talks of being responsible for her mother's death and says that she has something wrong inside her and needs an operation. She handles her baby roughly and shows little interest in it.

Questions

1. What is the probable diagnosis in this patient?

2. What special clinical features may be found in puerperal psychosis?

3. How common is mental disorder after childbirth?

4. What is the prospect for recovery in puerperal psychosis and the risk of recurrence with subsequent childbirth?

5. What etiological factors may be of importance in puerperal psychosis?

6. What is 'post-partum blues'?

7. How would you treat this patient?

Answers

Q1.

Since the illness involves psychotic features and has occurred within the puerperium it is, by definition, a puerperal psychosis but it is necessary to identify the particular diagnostic category i.e. organic, affective or schizophrenic. In this case the paranoid ideas, formal thought disorder of schizophrenic type and incongruity of affect would all suggest a schizophrenic illness but the presence at times of depressed mood and of depressive thought content (e.g. being responsible for her mother's death) point to a significant affective element and this may justify and initial diagnosis of a schizo-affective illness.

Q2.

Although psychiatric disorders arising in the puerperium resemble those occurring at any other time, certain features have been claimed to be characteristic though they may also be found in post-operative psychosis. These include, as in this case, the presence of confusion in the early stages of a functional disorder (affective or schizo-phrenic) despite the absence of any organic cause such as infection (before the advent of antibiotics acute organic mental states due to post-partum infection were relatively common) and an admixture of affective and schizophrenic symptomatology. A tendency to relapse after apparent recovery has also been described.

Q3.

The incidence of poset-partum psychosis that requires admission to a psychiatric unit is probably of the order of 1 to 500 births but milder disturbance is much commoner with about 10 per cent of women developing a significant degree of depression – usually after returning home from hospital. The peak incidence occurs during the first two weeks after delivery (apart from an immediate latency period of two days) but there is an increased psychiatric admission rate throughout the first three months post-partum.

Q4.

The prognosis for a puerperal illness is generally thought to be rather better than for the same condition occurring outside the puerperium. Figures for the likelihood of recurrence with further childbirth vary but suggest that the risk, i.e. the proportion of women who do have a subsequent puerperal psychosis, is of the order of 15 to 20 per cent. The incidence of subsequent non-puerperal psychosis may, however, be as high as 50 per cent.

Q5.

The view that post-partum psychosis is not a specific entity but is due to childbirth precipitating one of the psychoses in a predisposed individual is supported by their similarity to non-puerperal psychotics in terms of heredity, past psychiatric history and premorbid personality. There is a tendency for women who develop a puerperal psychosis to be primipara and a little older than normal puerperal controls. The role of hormonal changes has been considered, particularly because of the frequency of a history of premenstrual tension and the usual 'latency period' between delivery and the onset of the illness, but with little convincing evidence and hormones seem to have no part to play in treatment. Psychological factors have also been claimed to be important — supported by the existence of 'adoption psychosis' and 'puerperal psychoses' in husbands. Marital discord and a state of conflict over the coming birth is often postulated in such theories and certainly unplanned pregnancy appears to be a risk factor but so also is death of the baby around the time of birth (as in the case of this patient's sister).

Q6.

The relationship of 'post-partum blues' to clinical depression is unclear. It is possibly related to decreased tryptophan turnover and affects about $\frac{2}{3}$ of women. It is transient and usually clears up without psychiatric intervention, however 10 per cent of those affected may develop clinical depression.

Q7.

A patient with a post-partum illness of this severity should be treated in a psychiatric unit but with facilities for the admission of the baby in order to enable 'bonding' — the formation of the normal mother-infant relationship. As far as possible the patient should be allowed, under supervision, to maintain contact with her baby and to care for it. Breast feeding may be continued though the possibility of psychotropic drugs given to the patient being present in the milk and thus ingested by the baby must be borne in mind. Treatment of the psychosis should not differ from that appropriate for the same condition occurring outside the puerperium. In this case, since there is a mixture of affective and schizophrenic symptomatology, both antidepressants for the former and neuroleptics for the latter would be appropriate. ECT might also be considered if progress proved slow. As soon as improvement allows she should go home for weekends with the baby with a view to early discharge though sudden relapse has to be watched for.

Course and management

This patient's course in hospital was very variable both in terms of symptomatology and overall level of disturbance with more than one relapse after apparent improvement. Because of the schizophrenic symptomatology she was treated with chlorpromazine, trifluoperazine and, later, depot injections of flupenthixol. Depressive features became more prominent however and she had ECT with improvement, relapse and then further improvement. At one stage she was discharged after apparent recovery and a good weekend at home only to be readmitted two days later in a depressed state for which she was prescribed amitriptyline. She remained agitated and paranoid and had to be detained under Section 25 of the Mental Health Act after walking out twice. After this her mood gradually changed and she became overactive, garrulous and hypomanic. At this stage the flupenthixol injection was changed to fluphenazine (as more sedative) and she was started on lithium because of the bipolar nature of the affective disturbance. With this medication she improved and was discharged after a total admission of about five months. The final diagnosis was of a puerperal psychosis of schizoaffective type and she was to continue on lithium, fluphenazine, trifluoperazine, orphenadrine and amitriptyline.

Further reading

Dean C, Kendell R E 1981 The symptomatology of puerperal illnesses. Brit J Psychiat 139: 128–133

Pitt B 1975 Psychiatric illness following childbirth. In: Silverstone T, Barraclough B (eds) Contemporary Psychiatry, Headly Bros Ltd

Protheroe C 1969 Puerperal psychoses: a long term study 1927–1961. Brit J Psychiat 115: 9–30

Tod E D M 1964 Lancet 2: 1264

CASE 57

A charge nurse directs the attention of the ward doctor to a 60-year-old male chronic schizophrenic patient whom he thinks is depressed. The patient is informal and has spent over 40 years in institutions and little is known about his family background or early years. When first admitted to hospital he was described as 'odd in manner, detached from reality and preoccupied with his own thoughts. He stares out of the window, shows little interest in his surroundings, his speech is hesitant and inappropriate. He has delusions of persecution and grandeur, and is roused to anger without adequate cause'. He is thought to be homosexually orientated, but this has never been a problem for him. He worked in various hospitals as a gardener, but was never considered well enough for discharge. He enjoys his work and visits the patients' social centre. In the preceding two weeks it was noticed that he was 'reluctant to go out of the ward, has become withdrawn and less social'. His interest in watching television has declined, and he has become less active around the ward. His appetite has also declined, but his sleep is apparently undisturbed and he has not complained of depression. At interview the patient looks depressed, and answers 'yes' when asked he does not welcome the interview. He denies perceptual disturbance and indeed there is no clear cut evidence of positive or negative symptoms of schizophrenia. General physical examination is negative, but he has two large inguinal herniae and these are described as 'giving him increasing discomfort' over the preceding two years. He has adamantly refused to have a surgical opinion or wear a truss, and he is not on medication.

Questions

1. What is your formulation on this patient?

2. How is the course of schizophrenia influenced by the emotional atmosphere in the home?

3. What do you know of monosymptomatic delusional psychosis?

4. Briefly how would you classify anti-psychotic drugs other than lithium?

5. How frequently is depression encountered in schizophrenia?

6. What is meant by 'positive and negative symptoms of schizophrenia'?

7. How would you manage this patient?

8. If this patient considered his homosexaul orientation a burden
and requested treatment, which treatments are available?

9. Would you compulsorily submit this patient to a surgical opinion or treatment of his herniae?

Answers

Q1.

This 60-year-old male patient, described as a 'chronic schizophrenic' with a duration of hospitalisation of about 40 years, is
probably at present suffering from endogenous depression. This is
characterised by a subjective feeling of depression, generalised psychomotor retardation, with low interest in his daily activities and
his surroundings and without an obvious precipitant. His presentation is probably coloured by institutionalisation and a deficit effect
of schizophrenia, although he is without clear cut positive or negative symptoms of schizophrenia at present. Antidepressant treatment is indicated.

Q2.

There is now considerable evidence that the course of schizophrenia
is influenced by the emotional atmosphere generated in the home
by the patient's key relatives. It has been demonstrated that the
relapse rate over a nine month period is twice as high for patients
returning to high expressed emotion 'E.E.' homes as for patients
returning to low 'E.E.' homes. Psychophysiological measurements
of arousal have been performed on patients in high and in low 'E.E.'
homes during the presence and the absence of key relatives and
significant differences were noted between the two patient groups.
Patients in low 'E.E.' homes rapidly habituate to the presence of
a key relative so that their state of arousal declined over a period.
Patients from high 'E.E.' homes did not acclimatize and remained
in a state of high arousal during the presence of the key relative.
It has not been fully established that these psychophysiological
responses to high 'E.E.' is peculiar to schizophrenia or will not tend
to induce relapse in other psychiatric conditions. It is of course well

established that stressful social interactions will produce a state of high arousal and it has been noted that stressful situations and major life events frequently occur in the weeks and months prior to schizophrenic relapse. The associations between high 'E.E'. relatives, high arousal in schizophrenic patients and the tendency to relapse have not been fully established as causal; studies to establish this are in progress.

Q3.

A delusion presenting as a solitary symptom is encountered in a small percentage of patients. The solitary encapsulated delusion is often of a hypochondriacal nature. A delusion concerning the functioning of the gastro-intestinal tract is the most common and the patient may first attend a dentist or a gastro-enterologist for help. They may complain of a foul smell from the mouth, or the anus, or that the bowels are rotting or blocked. The personality structure is intact and no other psychiatric symptomatology is evident. It may have a very disruptive effect on the patient's life and up to recently was intractable to treatment, and frequently resulted in unnecessary investigations and surgical treatment. More recently reports in the literature claimed success in treatment with behavioural psychotherapy, and also with pimozide. Its precise relationship to schizophrenia is unclear but it may be observed in chronic schizophrenic patients who otherwise have been symptomatically quiescent for years.

Q4.

Antipsychotic drugs can be classified chemically into phenothiazines, butyrophenones, phenylbutilpiperidines and thioxanthines. There is considerable overlap in their indications and they share many anticholinergic and extrapyramidial side effects. The phenothiazines are the most widely used and they can be divided into three main groups, on the basis of the strength of their sedative action and side effects. In the first group are chlorpromazine which could be regarded as the prototype of all the phenothiazines and promazine. These have pronounced sedative effects and moderate anticholinergic and extrapyramidal side effects. Chlorpromazine has of course been extensively used in the treatment of schizophrenia. The second group of phenothiazines is comprised of pericyazine and thioridazine. These drugs have moderate sedative effects, marked anticholinergic effects and minimal extrapyramidal side effects. Thioridazine due to its minimal extrapyramidal side effects has been extensively prescribed as a tranquilliser in the elderly. The third group of phenothiazines is comprised of such drugs as perphena-

zine, fluphenazine and trifluoperazine. These drugs are characterised by minimal anticholinergic effects and pronounced
extrapyramidal side effects. A direct antipsychotic effect is claimed
for some of these preparations. Trifluoperazine is commonly prescribed for schizophrenic patients with florid symptomatology. The
butyrophenones include droperidol, haloperidol and trifluperidol,
they have minimal anticholinergic effects and marked extrapyramidal side effects. They have been used principally to control the
symptoms of mania and hypomania. The piperidol group is comprised of fluspirilene and pimozide and drugs in this group also have
minimal anticholinergic effects but may have extrapyramidal side
effects. These drugs are used in the treatment of schizophrenia and
related psychoses. Fluspirilene is administered in the form of a long
acting intra-muscular preparation. The last major group of antipsychotic drugs is the thioxanthine group comprised of clopenthixol,
flupenthixol and thiothixene, these are less sedating than chlorpromazine and extrapyramidal symptoms are more frequent, they
are claimed to be beneficial in schizophrenic patients with negative
symptoms such as apathy and withdrawal and flupenthixol is available as a depot injection.

Q5.
Depression is frequently encountered in all stages of a schizophrenic illness. In one study $\frac{1}{2}$ of untreated new acute schizophrenics and $\frac{1}{3}$ of chronic schizophrenics who relapsed whether treated
or not were found to be depressed. It has been observed in another
study that more schizophrenic patients required inpatient treatment
for depression than for relapse of their illness. The relationship
between neuroleptic drugs and depression in the setting of schizophrenia is unclear. The prevalence of depression in drug-free patients
both for first illness and relapsed schizophrenia is high. Some
depressive symptoms may be drug related or dose related as it has
been observed that both high dose of medication and the development of drug induced extrapyramidal symptoms correlate at a level
of significance with the presence of depression. However, it has also
been noted that patients maintained in remission on regular depot
injections had the lowest prevalence of depression. Although there
are many theories on why depression is commonly encountered in
schizophrenia, the question will only be resolved when we know
much more of the etiological and phenomenological relationship of
affective psychosis to the schizophreniform psychoses.

Q6.
The positive symptoms of schizophrenia could be described as

abnormal psychological features such as delusions, hallucinations and thought disorder and the negative symptoms as diminished or absent normal functions such as poverty of speech, flattening of affect, loss of volition, withdrawal and apathy. Considerable discussion exists on the nosological and prognostic significance of these symptoms. Bleuler and Kraepelin emphasised the importance of the negative symptoms for diagnosis and prognosis of schizophrenia. In brief they regarded the presence of negative symptoms as fundamental to the diagnosis and the prognosis was poor broadly in direct relationship to the marked presence of these symptoms. Many years later Schneider advocated his 'first rank' symptoms as pathognomonic of schizophrenia. These symptoms were regarded as 'positive' because they were more easily identifiable and rateable. The main criticism of Schneider's symptoms is that they are of poor prognostic value as many chronic schizophrenic patients are not known to have had them. Kraepelin and Bleuler recognised these symptoms but regarded them as epi-phenomena or variable accompaniments of schizophrenia. At present considerable discussion exists on the significance of positive and negative symptoms. The terms type I syndrome has been used for an illness with positive symptoms and type II syndrome for an illness with negative symptoms. As acute schizophrenia frequently presents with positive symptoms (type I) and tends to respond to neuroleptic medication and chronic schizophrenia presents with negative symptoms (type II) and has a poor prognosis irrespective of drug treatment, separate disease dimensions or different pathological processes have been postulated for each of the two types. The suggestion is that the two types can be understood as disturbances along a single continuum of instability in the control of dopaminergic transmission. According to this view under-activity of dopaminergic transmission is reflected as negative symptoms and superimposed episodes of over-activity as positive symptoms. However, the observation that positive and negative symptoms may occur simultaneously is not easy to reconcile with this theory. The view that there are different underlying pathological processes is based on the observations that the positive symptoms of acute schizophrenia (not the negative ones) respond to neuroleptic medication. Some chronic schizophrenic patients with negative symptoms show C.T. scan evidence of increased ventricular size. Type II syndrome is also associated with nerve cell loss and type I syndrome with an increased number of dopamine receptors. However, even if type I and type II have different underlying pathological processes, this does not necessarily mean that the processes are unrelated or that the two syndromes represent separate diseases. The discussion and the research continues.

Q7.
This patient should receive a course of tricyclic or tetracyclic anti-depressants and their effect should be monitored over a two to three week period. If he is unresponsive to one, another should be tried. As the patient is rather miserable, and E.C.T. may be quickly effective, there should not be undue delay in awaiting a response to antidepressants, before prescribing E.C.T. The prognosis for his depression is probably good.

Q8.
Very few patients with an exclusive homosexual orientation will seek treatment for it. Those who seek treatment are likely to be incidentally homosexual and worried about their difficulty in obtaining partners, the animosity of others towards them and increasing loneliness and isolation. The object of treatment is to re-orientate or suppress their sexual inclination. Dynamic and behavioural forms of psychotherapy are methods of treatment in use. In general, the higher the homosexual tendency in the Kinsey ratings, (that is the more exclusive the tendency) the less likelihood there is of success in treatment. Results of treatment with dynamic psychotherapy differ and range from 0 to 50 per cent success. The groups studied may not have been comparable and may have had different Kinsey ratings. Success rates of 40 per cent have been claimed for behavioural techniques. Aversion techniques by pairing deviant material with mild electric shocks or apomorphine-induced nausea is the commonest behavioural treatment used. Chemical and electrical methods appear to be equally effective, but electrical methods due to convenience are more frequently used. Homosexuals, in general, do not respond to treatment as well as other sexual deviationists such as fetishists, bisexuals and transvestites. If the sexual deviation is associated with anti-social behaviour such as violence then an anti-androgen drug with minimal feminising effects, may be used. Cyproterone which is reputed to reduce both desire and potency has been widely used.

Q9.
I would not compulsorily submit this informal patient for a surgical opinion or treatment. Although his herniae are probably causing discomfort, they are present over a long period of time and are not at present presenting an immediate or serious threat to life and his wish not to have treatment should be respected. The patient should be encouraged to seek treatment and if a complication such as stran-

gulation developed then of course compulsory surgical intervention
may be unavoidable.

Course and management

The patient responded to amitriptyline 50 mg t.d.s. after about two
weeks. He resumed his daily activities and continued with the
antidepressant.

Further reading

Beary M D, Cobb J P 1981 Solitary psychosis — three cases of monosymptomatic
  delusion of alimentary stench treated with behavioural psychotherapy. Brit J
  Psychiat 138: 64–66

Freeman T 1982 Positive and negative schizophrenic symptoms. Correspondence.
  Brit J Psychiat 140: 210–211

Johnson D A W 1981 Studies of depressive symptoms in schizophrenia. The
  prevalence of depression and its possible causes. Brit J Psychiat 139: 89–93

Leff J, Vaughn C 1981 The role of maintenance therapy and relatives' expressed
  emotion in relapse of schizophrenia. A two year follow up. Brit J Psychiat 139:
  102–104

MacKay A V P, Crow T J 1980 A discussion — positive and negative
  schizophrenia symptoms and the role of dopamine. Brit J Psychiat 137:
  379–386

Case Index

Subject Index